A c
Do

D0242207

A career in medicine: Do you have what it takes?

SECOND EDITION

Edited by
Rameen Shakur MPhil (Cantab)

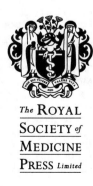

The ROYAL
SOCIETY of
MEDICINE
PRESS Limited

British Library Cataloguing in Publication Data
A catalogue record for this book is available from the British Library
ISBN 1-85315-633-7
ISBN 978-1-85315-633-5

Distribution in Europe and Rest of World:
Marston Book Services Ltd
PO Box 269
Abingdon
Oxon OX14 4YN, UK
Tel: +44 (0)1235 465500
Fax: +44 (0)1235 465555
Email: direct.order@marston.co.uk

Distribution in the USA and Canada:
Royal Society of Medicine Press Ltd
c/o BookMasters Inc
30 Amberwood Parkway
Ashland, OH 44805, USA
Tel: +1 800 247 6553/+1 800 266 5564
Fax: +1 419 281 6883
Email: order@bookmasters.com

Distribution in Australia and New Zealand:
Elsevier Australia
30–52 Smidmore Street
Marrikville NSW 2204, Australia
Tel: +61 2 9517 8999
Fax: +61 2 9517 2249
Email: service@elsevier.com.au

Typeset by Phoenix Photosetting, Chatham, Kent
Printed in Great Britain by
Creative Print & Design (Wales), Ebbw Vale

Contributors

Editor

Dr Rameen Shakur F2 Academic Medicine Rotation: Cardiology. Nuffield Department of Medicine, the John Radcliffe Hospital, University of Oxford

Authors

Dr Kamran Abbasi Editor, Journal of the Royal Society of Medicine, London

Dr Yasir Al-Wakeel F2 Academic Medicine Rotation. Nuffield Department of Medicine, the John Radcliffe Hospital, University of Oxford

Dr Paul Ayuk Former Clinical Lecturer in Obstetrics and Gynaecology, the John Radcliffe Hospital, University of Oxford

Professor Raanan Gillon Emeritus Professor of Medical Ethics, Imperial College of Science, Technology and Medicine, London

Mr Ashok Handa Honorary Consultant Vascular Surgeon and Clinical Tutor in Surgery, Nuffield department of Surgery, the John Radcliffe Hospital, University of Oxford

Dr Hywel Jones District Clinical Tutor, the John Radcliffe Hospital, University of Oxford

Abhishek Joshi Graduate Medical Student, University of Oxford

Stuart Laverack Final Year Medical Student, University of Sheffield

Kirsty Lloyd Chair, BMA Medical Students Committee

Dilshad Marikhar Graduate Medical Student, St George's Medical School, London

Andrew Pearson Former Finance Chair, BMA Medical Students Committee

Dr Faheem Shakur F1 Houseman, General Medicine, The Royal Preston Hospital, Preston, Lancs

Dr Edward Shaoul Honorary Senior Lecturer, Imperial College London

Professor John Stein Medical Admissions Tutor, Magdalen College, University of Oxford

Emily Stobbs Medical Student, University of Nottingham

Dr Simon Thorn Head of Biology, Radley College, Oxfordshire

Professor Robin Williamson Professor of Surgery, imperial College London, Consultant Surgeon, Hammersmith Hospital and former Dean, the Royal Society of Medicine, London

About the editor

Dr Rameen Shakur is a 25-year-old Cambridge and Edinburgh (clinical) University graduate currently undertaking a Foundation Year 2 (F2) academic medical rotation in Cardiology at the NDM (Nuffield Department of Medicine), the John Radcliffe Hospital, Oxford. He is a Clinical Tutor in General Surgery at the Nuffield Department of Surgery and a Clinical Teacher in Medicine for Green and Worcester Colleges at the University of Oxford.

He has won numerous prizes and scholarships, most notably a Churchill Fellowship for Harvard Medical School for the application of genomic medicine in Cardiology, a Peter Kirk Fellowship, a Wellcome Trust scholarship for the Sanger Centre Genome Campus, Cambridge and a British Heart Foundation grant for cardiovascular research as a medical student. His hobbies include playing cricket, football and listening to Indian classical music.

He studied at Hutton Grammar School and Sixth-Form, Preston, Lancashire. His research interests include molecular cardiology, immunological markers of disease and transplantation rejection.

Contents

Foreword

I am delighted that a second edition of this book has been published. The first edition, which I edited in 2000, was the child of a study day which was developed at the Royal Society of Medicine for sixth form students. The book was popular enough to be reprinted twice in 2003 as it met a need – namely to clothe the dream of a medical career with the reality of achieving that goal.

The criteria for student selection are changing, as are the methods of teaching and learning. Even in the last few years, the expectations of the public and the work pattern of doctors have changed. Anyone considering a career in medicine must be aware of these developments. These changes and the established ways of the profession are addressed in the new edition, which will be invaluable to all those considering becoming a doctor.

It is good to see that the wisdom and experience of some of the original contributors, which has stood the test of time, is retained. There are welcome new chapters, such as those on the historical background to modern medicine, student finance, academic medicine and medical journalism, which broaden the scope and appeal of the book.

The second edition is a more than worthy successor to the first. In addition to supplementing the study day at the Royal Society of Medicine, it will stand alone as an essential part of informed decision making for those considering a career in medicine.

Harvey White

Preface

Life is short, the art long, opportunity fleeting, experiment treacherous, judgement difficult.

Hippocrates

Making independent and informed decisions is one of the harder tasks in life. Some of the decisions you have to make can affect your own future, your livelihood and even the future of your family. Choosing the right career is one such decision, and so adequate time and effort on formulating a realistic and informed choice is important, especially so if that career is to be in medicine.

Numerous students have found the information in the first edition of this book very useful in formulating a realistic picture of a life in medicine and the application process involved. However, given recent changes in school and medical curricula, the introduction of more graduate entry schemes and the ongoing financial concerns facing all university students, it was time to update the book.

This edition has been researched thoroughly to incorporate the most recent changes to medical careers as announced by the government through the Modernising Medical Careers committee.

Also, for the first time, chapters relating to academic medicine, careers in medical journalism, graduate entry and medical student funding have been included, alongside updated versions of the chapters that had made the book a clear favourite among students in the past. The second edition continues the tradition of the first in providing independent, concise and thorough information relating to aspects of a career in medicine and how to achieve this goal.

We envisage this book to be of great value not only for candidates who are thinking about entering medical school, but also for current medical students and junior doctors alike. Please visit the website which accompanies the book for more information on aspects of the book's content: www.acareerinmedicine.net.

Rameen Shakur
Oxford, 2006

Acknowledgements

This book has required much effort on the part of the contributors and the RSM Press staff. I would like to thank all of the contributors for their time and effort in producing their chapters and for researching their topics so thoroughly. I would like to thank in particular Harvey White, who gave me this opportunity after the great success of the first edition. A very big thanks should also go to Peter, Ian, Hannah and Laura from RSM Press for their support and hard work during the production of the book.

Thank you also to all my colleagues at the John Radcliffe Hospital for their support during the writing of this book, namely Dr AKM Muktadir, Dr Dalia Wahab, Dr Hywel Jones, Dr David Holdsworth, Dr David Nasralla, Mr Ashok Handa, all the staff of the Postgraduate Centre at the John Radcliffe, and my consultants Professor Warrell, Dr Dwight and Professor Becker.

Finally, I would like to thank my family – my mother, father and brother – for their unabated love and support during the whole of my student life. They have been inspirational in my development. I would like to say a big thank you to my mother and father for instilling my thirst for knowledge and my passion to ask the question, why?

I would like to dedicate this book to my grandparents (Abdul Wazid and Abdus Shakur), neither of whom are here to read this book, but were it not for their blessings, this and all my achievements thus far would not have come to fruition.

Medicine: Remembering the past, looking to the future

Abhishek Joshi, Graduate Entry Medical Student, University of Oxford
Dr Rameen Shakur, F2 Academic Medicine Rotation: Cardiology. Nuffield Department of Medicine, the John Radcliffe Hospital, University of Oxford

Doctors practising today can call on a huge body of knowledge and experience when they treat their patients. There are thousands of journals to read, hundreds of guidelines to follow and an almost unlimited number of scientific ideas to be used. Practising as a doctor involves applying new scientific discoveries and inventions to some old problems.

Yet it was not always like this. Every time a doctor takes a blood sample or listens to a patient's heart, he or she is utilizing thousands of years of thought, experiment and experience. There have been doctors, or people like them, for thousands of years, but their methods have been evolving and only very recently have they started to use the techniques that we are familiar with. The first doctors knew nothing about cells, organs or drugs. You might very well wonder how they managed to treat people at all, but they did. This chapter explores some of the major historical advances in medicine and those that helped shape the ethos of medical practice.

The spirit of medicine

Much of modern Western medicine stems from the ancient Greeks, where the main practitioners of medicine were priests. The ancient Greeks originally thought that diseases were caused by the gods deciding to punish the patient. The treatment was prayer, and many priests would prescribe patients potions that would make them enter a state of shock. The idea was that a god could then appear before them and they could ask to be made well again. Medicine was closely associated with magic in the very early days, and the Greeks used combinations of 'magic numbers' in their treatment of diseases. For example, patients who were ill were quarantined for 40 days, because the number 40 was considered to be magical!

The idea that illness is some sort of punishment from God or the gods, and that it can be cured by prayer and ritual continues today. In fact, some scientists are now engaged in researching whether prayer actually works to improve people's health.

Hippocrates

After a while, the Greeks began to think differently about the world around them, and also about disease and health. In particular, Hippocrates (460–377BC) introduced a number of new ideas, and is now known as the 'Father of Medicine'. Hippocrates taught his medical students how to recognize the outward features of disease, and encouraged them to learn which features suggested the severity of the disease. This brought about the idea that doctors could make a diagnosis and a prognosis for a person based on observation, and helped Greek doctors to begin to classify illnesses.

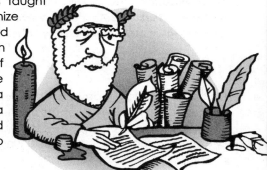

Hippocrates also popularized the idea of the 'humours' in medicine. The Greek theory of the humours was that everything in the world was made up from a combination of the four elements: air, water, fire and earth. Hippocrates associated these elements with humours (or fluids) in the body: air with blood, green bile with fire, black bile with earth, and phlegm with water. He believed that if someone had too much of one of these humours, the resulting imbalance, or *dyscrasia*, caused illness. The obvious cure, then, would be to remove some of the humour, so he suggested sneezing or vomiting as cures for diseases. Interestingly, Hippocrates also believed that doctors should try to do as little as possible and let the patient recover naturally.

These theories of humours are 'holistic', in that they treat the energies of the person rather than the specific disease, but people like Hippocrates did begin to recognize the importance of individual organs in the body, suggesting that they had a role in producing the different humours. Hippocrates was also credited with writing the Hippocratic oath, the ethical code of conduct that doctors swear to follow, although a number of similar oaths existed before his time. Interestingly, the Hippocratic oath separates doctors from surgeons, as surgeons were considered uneducated servants of the doctors.

Ayurvedic medicine

The idea that illness was characterized by an imbalance in the patients' elements was not exclusive to the Greeks.

Early Indians practised the Ayurvedic method of medicine over 3000 years ago, and the practice still survives in India today, often allied to modern 'biomedical' practice.

The system teaches doctors to maintain a balance between the five elements of ether, air, water, fire and earth. Early Hindus believed that the knowledge of Ayurvedic medicine came directly from the god Brahma, and the main texts were the *Charaka* and the *Sushrata*, which were written down after a period of word-of-mouth. The system is very complex, and divides the mind, body and soul into separate systems. There are detailed explanations of how disease occurs and specific medicines for each disease, aimed at restoring the patient's balance. Ayurvedic physicians had to learn eight different disciplines: internal medicine; surgery and anatomy; eye, ear, nose and throat diseases; paediatrics (and embryology); demonology (or psychiatry); toxicology; rejuvenation; and fertility.

In addition, the physician would have to master the study of chemistry, so he could make his own medicines, which were usually made from plants. Training took seven years, and at the end doctors were required to take an oath promising to put their patient's care above all else.

The Egyptians

Hippocrates' teaching remained popular in ancient Greece, and was refined over generations. As Alexander the Great spread his influence across the Mediterranean, his scholars took the Hippocratic model with them. When the great library of Alexandria was founded in Egypt, the Greek methods met with the (much older) Egyptian doctrines. This meeting was particularly fruitful.

The Egyptian method of practising medicine dates back to 3000BC. The Egyptians, too, believed that illness was due to the influence of gods and spirits, and they used an array of potions and spells to heal their patients. The Egyptians worshipped one of the first royal physicians, Imhotep, as the god of healing. Imhotep wrote what has become known as the 'Edwin Smith Papyrus'. This documents, in exquisite detail, the Egyptian methods for examination, diagnosis, treatment and prognosis of a number of diseases. The Egyptians were also aware of public health, and by 1150BC (the 19th Dynasty), they were providing medical insurance and sick leave for workers building the pyramids.

The crucial difference between the Greeks and the Egyptians was in their study of anatomy. Whereas the Greeks considered the body sacred and so did not dissect cadavers, the Egyptians dissected cadavers as a matter of course. This led to a better understanding of human anatomy. The Egyptian understanding allowed surgical practice to develop, and the Egyptians also had a better understanding of things such as the pulse and the functions of different organs.

Some scholars at the school in Alexandria attempted to use an empirical approach to medicine. This meant that they listened to the patient's complaint (a history), examined the patient and then made a diagnosis – just as doctors do today.

The problem was that these doctors did not understand the diseases they were studying well enough to relate the symptoms and signs to a disease, and when they could, they did not know what to do about it. This meant that the perfectly rational idea was out-competed by the 'methodic' school, who were obsessed with the state of patients' pores. This school of doctors thought that the pores on the skin were a direct reflection of the patient's health, and so they suggested a number of ways in which a person should wash in order to maintain healthy, open pores. The theory was popular because doctors could see the direct results of their treatments, even if they did not actually cure any diseases.

The Romans

As the Roman Empire began to take its hold in the 1st century AD and the Greeks became poorer, many Greek doctors continued to ply their trade as Roman slaves. Being a doctor in Rome was seen as a socially un-desirable job. However, a number of doctors were successful and were able to buy their freedom. One of the most successful Roman doctors was Galen (AD129–200), who was the son of a wealthy architect. He was never a slave, but instead studied at Alexandria, where he learned the Hippocratic theories of medicine, which he then brought to Rome. He developed these ideas and furthered the study of anatomy through public dissections of pigs and Barbary apes, which he considered to be anatomically similar to humans. He showed that the kidneys produced urine and demonstrated the importance of the spinal cord, but despite these useful experimental findings, Galen's effect on medicine was effectively to halt any real progress for over a thousand years after his death.

Galen recognized the importance of blood in sustaining the body, but thought that it was produced by the liver and then consumed by the rest of the body. He thought that blood was given a 'natural spirit' in the liver, a 'vital spirit' in the heart and an 'animal spirit' in the brain. Blood was then supposed to travel through the nerves to nourish the rest of the body with its spirits. The theory's flaw was not so much that it was inaccurate, as that it unfortunately fitted so well with the Christian ideas of the time. This meant that Galen's theories were promoted and protected by the Church in Europe, which ensured that his anatomical findings and theory of medicine were not challenged for over a thousand years. For example, people believed that the humerus bone in the arm was curved because Galen said so, and dismissed the straight bones they saw as 'tricks of nature'.

Galen's teachings thus survived virtually unchanged well into the 17th century. The main change over this time was the introduction of patron saints for each disease. These saints were petitioned for cures, in a return to the earlier ideas and superstitions that God or spirits intervened in man's health. For example, St Fiacre was supposed to protect the patient from haemorrhoids. There were few practical advances – medicine had entered the Dark Ages in Europe.

The Middle East

While European medicine had come to a virtual standstill, the Arabic world began to flourish. In the 6th century AD, King Khusraw of Persia began to welcome Christian refugees from the Byzantine Empire in the West and scholars from India and China in the East to Gondeshapur (in modern-day Iran). There they translated their texts and shared their accumulated knowledge, founding the first medical school. This cross-pollination of medical cultures allowed students in Gondeshapur to combine the different strands of medicine and to develop their ideas further, which provided fertile ground for the development of a number of eminent Middle Eastern medics.

Al-Razi (865–925) and Ibn Sina (Avicenna) (980–1037) were two major Arabic physicians, who wrote over 600 books between them. They both studied medicine alongside philosophy, mathematics, and other sciences and arts, and are credited with keeping the tradition of rational thought and discovery in medicine alive. Most of their work found its way to Europe, where it formed the basis of medical teaching.

Al-Razi lived in what is now Tehran in Iran. Despite being strongly influenced by the Hippocratic way of thinking, he described the symptoms and signs of diseases and did not try to explain them in terms of spirits or humours. He wrote about the diseases of smallpox and measles, and was careful to mark the differences between them. He relied on rational thought and observation, and this helped him make his discoveries. He also began to publish the first doubts about some of Galen's teachings.

Ibn Sina qualified as a doctor by the age of 18, and came to live in Tehran as the court doctor to the emir (king). He wrote almost constantly, and consolidated everything he knew about medicine (which in those days was considered to be everything there *was* to know about medicine) into a 14-volume book called *Canon of Medicine*. Ibn Sina built on the teachings of Galen and Al-Razi, and added his own experiences to his work. His book describes many diseases and what he thought caused them. He also described the functions of the various organs. In addition, he suggested that tuberculosis is infectious (something that European scholars disagreed with) and gave a clear account of the symptoms and complications of diabetes. The *Canon* was translated and distributed around Europe, and became the standard medical textbook for the next 700 years.

The Renaissance

Although progress in Europe was much slower compared with the golden era of the Middle East, this does not mean that nothing was happening in the field of medicine. The study of anatomy was progressing, not due to the work of doctors, but because of the work of artists such as Leonardo da Vinci (1452–1519). Da Vinci was interested in the human form from an artistic viewpoint, but soon began to study anatomy in a more systematic way. He was allowed to dissect corpses in the hospitals of Florence, Rome and Milan, despite the disapproval of the Church. These dissections led to some of the first accurate representations of human anatomy in Europe. Da Vinci described the skeleton, the skull, the positions of the organs and the attachments of the muscles. He discovered that the heart had four chambers, and had planned to publish all of his anatomical drawings, but died before he could do so.

Also working in Renaissance Italy, Vesalius (1514–1564) picked up where da Vinci left off. He was the first physician to base his anatomical knowledge directly on his dissection work – a huge break from the prevailing tradition. Up to that point, the study of anatomy in medical circles had come from Galen's work and from philosophical discussion. Vesalius demonstrated that the internal organization of the body was the same in all people, and that the organs were real, solid objects and not just theoretical concepts. He introduced the idea to medicine that 'seeing is believing' into medicine. Unless he could prove something by looking at it, he did not believe it. He contributed much to the study of anatomy through publishing many of his drawings and studies, but his main contribution was to start to change the way in which physicians thought about their subject. Doctors were no longer supposed just to accept previous dogma: they were encouraged to investigate and experiment and to base their practice on objective, observed measurements. Medicine had ceased to be an art, and was becoming a science. The application of rational thought and experimentation, along with the encouraging new political atmosphere, allowed the birth of science during the Renaissance. A better understanding of anatomy gave clinical techniques such as percussion and auscultation more value, while inventions such as the microscope helped physicians to appreciate the cellular nature of the body.

The Modern Age

Despite all these advances in understanding, there were still very few actual cures for diseases, which made the practice of medicine look a little futile. However, the scientific method of investigation and discovery led to an explosion in the fields of biology, chemistry and physics and to the development of entirely new branches of science. Literally thousands of these discoveries have fed into medical practice. In the past 300 years, advances in medicine have come at a rapid rate.

Notable advances include the individual contributions to vaccination by Jenner (1749–1823) and Pasteur (1822–1895). Jenner, a British physician, noticed that milkmaids did not get smallpox, and thought that this was because they were exposed to cowpox, which is similar but not life-threatening. He created a vaccine made from the cowpox blisters and tested it on a young boy, James Phipps. Phipps became immune to smallpox, and some time after Jenner's death the British government began to offer free vaccinations. Smallpox was eradicated throughout the world in 1980.

Pasteur built on Jenner's work, and was able to produce weaker strains of the bacteria and fungi that caused other diseases. This allowed him to produce new vaccinations for rabies and for anthrax. The use of observation and experimentation had allowed doctors to prevent and finally eradicate a deadly infectious disease – a huge leap forward in medical practice.

Doctors could now prevent diseases, but it required another breakthrough before they could actually claim to be able to cure them. Alexander Fleming (1881–1955), another British scientist, accidentally discovered that some of the mould he found growing in his unwashed Petri dishes was able to inhibit the growth of bacteria. He isolated some chemicals from the fungus, and called them penicillums. He noted that they killed many different types of bacteria, but he could not make them in sufficient quantities to be of any use. During the Second World War, scientists working in Oxford, most notably Howard Florey (1898–1968) and Ernst Chain (1906–1979), developed a way to produce large quantities of pure penicillin, creating the first antibiotic. Suddenly, the world had a way of treating and curing many bacterial infections, revolutionizing medicine.

Many other hugely important advances have come since the advent of the scientific method in medical research. William Morton (1819–1868) demonstrated the first use of anaesthetics in surgery, building on work by a number of chemists. His work in Massachusetts General Hospital led to the development of painless operations, which allowed surgeons to perform longer and more complex procedures. Wilhelm Röntgen (1845–1923) noticed that the radiation from some new electrical devices allowed him to take pictures of the bones in his hands. He worked with other scientists and eventually received the first ever Nobel Prize in Physics in 1901 for his discovery of X-rays. Other advances in pharmacology, physiology and genetics have allowed medical science to develop at an enormous pace.

Back to the future

These individual contributions to modern medicine are important, but the truth is that medicine no longer relies on the work of individuals to progress. With improvements in communication over the past few hundred years – from the printing press to the Internet – and because of the spread of the scientific method, there are now literally thousands of people working to bring about the next medical advance. This explosion of knowledge allows us to target our drugs to specific diseases and to develop new surgical techniques. It allows us to eradicate some diseases altogether, and to reduce the severity of those we cannot currently cure. It also means that today's doctors have a lot more to learn about and remember than Hippocrates or Galen could ever have imagined.

Despite this, there are plenty of lessons to be learned from history that can help doctors today. The original art of diagnosing a disease still uses methods that date back to Egyptian times; the schools in Alexandria and Gondeshapur remind us that medicine progresses when we share our knowledge; and while Galen's and Hippocrates' ideas may seem a little odd to us, they should remind doctors to be ethical and thoughtful. The experiences of Ibn Sina and Al-Razi should remind us to use rational thought during the formulation of our diagnosis and treatment and that we are treating people with diseases, not just diseases themselves.

The progression of medicine through the years has relied upon the ability of people to change the way they think and to adapt and use new information. The only thing constant about medicine today, as it was in the past, is that it is always evolving.

Further reading

Magner LN. *A History of Medicine*, 2nd edn. New York: Marcel Dekker, 1992.

Porter R. *The Greatest Benefit to Mankind: A Medical History of Humanity from Antiquity to the Present*. London: HarperCollins, 1997.

Singer C, Underwood EA. *A Short History of Medicine*, 2nd edn. Oxford: Oxford University Press, 1962.

Wootton D. *Bad Medicine – Doctors Doing Harm Since Hippocrates*. Oxford: Oxford University Press, 2006.

Entry requirements to medical school

2

Professor John Stein, Medical Admissions Tutor, Magdalen College, University of Oxford

Should you study medicine?

Although this chapter is mainly aimed at helping you get a place at a medical school, the degree of your commitment to medicine is so important, not only for achieving this but also for dictating whether you will enjoy a career in medicine afterwards, that I make no apology for starting by asking you again to think carefully about whether you really want to study medicine at all. If, having examined yourself and your motivation thoroughly and honestly, the pros do *not* easily outweigh the cons of a medical career for you, then I earnestly entreat that you seriously consider another career.

The ideal doctor should be not only knowledgeable about the human body and its diseases, but also compassionate and sensitive to people's feelings and have a burning desire to help people. The aim being to make a positive difference to people's lives, the doctor should be highly dedicated and committed to medicine, be very hard-working and conscientious, and have the highest integrity. You will need to be reasonably intelligent, with a retentive memory and an enquiring mind. You should want to know how the body works – but also be an articulate and sensitive communicator with very high personal standards of morality. You will need to have great energy and good organizational abilities, and to be tolerant of fairly long hours and hard physical labour. In addition, you should be able to cope with sometimes horrible people and often horrifying emotional traumas.

Such saints do not of course exist in real life! But that is what we aspire to, and these ideals dictate what you should be looking for in yourself. The most important quality is therefore a liking for and an interest in people, even the difficult ones. You need to really enjoy interacting and empathizing with all ranks, shapes, cultures, classes and religions, even trying to understand and sympathize with the problems of those who try to insult and humiliate you.

The next important requirement is an interest in how the body works, because modern medicine consists of the exciting application of hard-won scientific knowledge to helping people to counteract the cruel hereditary, environmental, social (and just plain random) determinants of disease. Thus, you must be interested not only in how smoking causes lung cancer or how high blood pressure causes kidney problems, but also in why Native Americans are intolerant of alcohol and why low-income groups have a hugely increased burden of disease, not only for themselves, but, sadly, also to pass on to their unborn children.

Then you must be practical. Eliciting physical signs, feeling for an enlarged liver, listening to heart murmurs and testing muscle reflexes are as important for making a diagnosis and deciding upon an appropriate course of treatment as your background knowledge and listening to your patient's history and how he describes his symptoms. Moreover, if you specialize in subjects such as surgery, anaesthesia or modern interventional radiology, you will need to develop even greater practical skills. However, there is nothing more rewarding than perfecting these skills. I shall never forget the joy after several attempts that had been painful (to both me and the patients) of finally getting the hang of lumbar puncturing, popping the needle in with no distress to me or patient, and the clear cerebrospinal fluid flowing out, without the patient having even a headache afterwards.

Finally, you must enjoy a life of great variety. There is very little predictable routine in medicine, and there are frequent moments of great stress. You must not lose your head at such times. You will have no more than 3 or 4 minutes to restart the heart when your patient collapses with ventricular fibrillation; so you cannot afford your mind to go blank while you panic about what to do.

Medicine can be almost a 24-hour occupation; but the hours are far less demanding than they used to be. Nevertheless, you have to be flexible; heart attacks seldom conveniently resolve at 5 PM. It is also emotionally demanding, because you are in the privileged position of taking responsibility for other people's lives. In addition, the corollary of your compassionate and sensitive empathy with your patients may be a crushing sense of failure when they die, despite your best efforts.

For the first 10 years or so of your life in medicine, because you lack the experience that really counts, you may feel that you are at the bottom of a heavy hierarchy that can make you feel very small and undervalued. However, you speedily become a useful member, and respect for this professional teamwork is fast improving the status of junior doctors. On top of all this, the 5-year medical course is one of the longest and hardest-working undergraduate courses. Yet, do not forget that by the time you are fully qualified, you and the state will have spent close to £200 000 on your training, and at the end of it all you will be relatively well paid. Furthermore, you will be equipped to follow a huge range of further careers, from primary care through to brain surgery, from Harley Street to TB or HIV treatment in sub-Saharan Africa.

Work experience

You must be sure that for you the drawbacks of medicine do not outweigh its positives. How strong you judge the arguments in favour of a career in medicine really does depend on you, your experience and your character. To help you make up your mind, obtain as much information as you can about what medicine is really like – for example, by shadowing GPs or hospital doctors, by attending their clinics, or by voluntary help in hospitals. Telephone or write to your local hospital, asking for work experience. You may have to be persistent and call several hospitals, as many are understandably cautious about whom they let in. You have a better chance if you wait until you are over 16. Also ask your family doctor; he or she will usually be sympathetic. You may end up doing routine clerical duties, but grin and bear it – it will teach you much about medicine. Some pathologists will even allow sixth-form students to witness postmortems. Write to your local hospital and ask them.

Admissions tutors do realize that arranging medical shadowing for people under the age of 18 is becoming more and more difficult with the rise of 'risk assessments' and fear of litigation; so we are happy with you obtaining your experience of medicine at some degree of distance, for instance by hospital portering or helping out in old people's homes.

Get a part-time job in a care home or hospice. These are usually easy to come by, and show you to be a practical person who is not afraid to get her hands dirty. If there are not any paid vacancies, ask if you can volunteer. Hospices in particular are always looking for helpers. Take up any chances for voluntary work that you can, since almost anything is useful.

When you are on work experience, be prepared to help out with the most menial tasks, and try to be as pleasant and helpful as possible.

If you can, make a point of talking most to junior doctors, because they see medicine at its toughest. If you think you are going to be interested in doing medical research and academic medicine, in addition try to visit hospital or medical school laboratories to see what goes on in them. Almost anything you have done, especially activities that involve teamwork, will add to your experience and show that you are a well-rounded individual who can get on with others.

If at the end of all this you finally decide that being able to help people at their most vulnerable, making a difference to their lives, and contributing to life and death decisions, will suit you, you will find medicine infinitely rewarding and fulfilling, well worth the sacrifice of your time and effort. You will gain gratitude, respect, status and trust from your patients and your peers. Also, you will seldom be unemployed and your salary will be reasonably good and reliable. However, if you feel you may resent the time and effort that you will have to dedicate, and the way in which medicine can to some extent dominate your life, and you really want to earn very large amounts of money, maybe medicine is not your profession.

Getting a medical school place

After this thorough and honest weighing up of all the considerations, you are now convinced that you want to apply to read medicine. So now you must set about maximizing your chances of getting in. The first thing is to be realistic: it is competitive, but not so bad as it used to be. Currently, you have a 50% chance of getting in at present; about two people apply for each of the current 7000 places per year available at the 31 British medical schools. However, because each person has four choices, this can look far worse, so that the current favourite, Nottingham, has over 20 candidates applying for each place. How you choose which medical school to apply to is the subject of another chapter. However, to make your choices as well informed as possible, do visit as many medical schools as you can on their open days, and talk to the students there. They will give you the best idea of what the place is really like.

GCSEs

Now, you must begin to organize your school campaign to gain a place at medical school, starting as early as possible. You will need to get as many As and A*s at GCSE as you can. At present, your GCSEs are the only public examination results that selection panels have to judge you by. Also, they are known to predict university degree performance – in fact, rather better than A levels, since they are not so easy to cram for. So selectors pay a great deal of attention to GCSE results, and some medical schools even state that they will not consider anybody with less than four As at GCSE unless there are special circumstances. You will usually need to have passed at least Maths, Physics, Chemistry, Biology, English and a language other than English (e.g. Welsh, French, or Spanish). Remember that GCSE double science will usually substitute for Physics, Chemistry and Biology, but not for Maths. Remember also that most universities try to be flexible. So if your first language is not English, English can be your second language. Also, if you have had no chance to do a second language, many universities will waive that requirement.

UCAS form

Selectors will pay as much attention to your personal statement as to your examination record and school report. In your personal statement, try not to tell us standard things about why you want to be a doctor. Everyone says much the same thing. Instead, try to communicate to us your genuine personal interest in medicine and your desire to help people in trouble. You must demonstrate your energy and enthusiasm to become a doctor, and that you have thought about what medicine actually entails through work experience or other attachments. Try to distil your own personal conclusions from your experiences. We also like to see that you have a variety of other interests, not because oarsmen, actresses or pianists necessarily make better doctors, but because achieving any of these to a high standard at the same time as achieving academic success demonstrates your wider horizons, together with your ability to work in a team and to organize yourself sufficiently well to find time to do both. Practise putting all this down in several versions before committing yourself to the actual UCAS form.

Your school report should make the same points, reinforcing your account of your past and potential future achievements – academic, sporting, cultural, political or social. It should also provide further evidence of your having thought deeply about medicine as a career, by experiencing it at first hand through work experience. So find out who is going to write your reference, and make sure that he or she actually knows something about you. They must read and reinforce your personal statement by giving their own opinions and further evidence about how intelligent, energetic, enthusiastic, well organized and committed to a career in medicine you are.

AS and A2 levels

Of course, the main thing your school report will contain is your AS grades if you have cashed them in, and your school's predictions of your A-level or IB (International Baccalaureate) grades. Your final A2-level grades have to be a minimum of AAB or IB equivalent these days, unless there are very exceptional reasons for lower grades. As for the subjects you should take, for most medical schools practically the only essential is Chemistry as far as A2 level. This is because much of physiology, biochemistry, pharmacology and molecular pathology depend upon a good knowledge of chemical reactions and their mechanisms. One other science or Maths is usually required. Although currently East Anglia, Hull/York and Nottingham insist on Biology rather than Chemistry, A-level Biology is not essential at most medical schools, so long as you have taken it or double science at GCSE. Nevertheless, most aspiring medical students will probably take Biology at A level simply because they will find it interesting, particularly the human aspects.

Thus, if you have studied only the physical sciences and Maths at A level, you are also welcomed by most medical schools. Of course you must be seriously interested in medicine. One thing that this often means in practice is that in the interview you will be asked how you think your knowledge of the physical sciences will help you in your medical studies and thereafter. So you should have thought carefully and acquired some knowledge about how the subjects that you have studied do relate to medicine, for example by knowing something about magnetic resonance imaging or the use of radioactive isotopes in radiotherapy. Many very successful doctors did the physical sciences at A level, and they were not impeded at all by not having studied biology at that stage. We find that after a few weeks becoming familiar with the nomenclature of medical science, much of which is borrowed from biology, those who have studied the physical sciences progress just as fast as the biologists.

You will also have noticed that most medical schools now require only two sciences at A level. Some are even happy with only Chemistry. This means that if you want to take an arts subject at A level, this is encouraged by most medical schools and it will not disadvantage you in any way. This change has come about because we now emphasize much more the importance of doctors' ability to communicate successfully with their patients from all walks of life. Study of an arts subject should not only cultivate your literacy skills, but also broaden your mind to other cultures and classes, and other ways of thinking and communicating.

BMAT (Bio-Medical Admissions Test)

Oxford, Cambridge, University College London (UCL), Imperial College London (ICL) and Manchester medical schools now set another test for medical students in order to determine whom they will interview; only the top 50% are interviewed. BMAT consists of three parts: a commentary on an English passage about some current topic of biomedical interest; a test of scientific knowledge pitched no higher than the GCSE syllabuses in Biology, Physics and Chemistry; and a quantitative reasoning test, which often takes the form of interpreting what you can conclude from a graph of scientific or clinical data.

Gap year?

Most medical schools are now happy if you want to take a year between school and university to travel, so long as your proposed programme is constructive, visiting countries with interesting medical problems or doing a useful job, not lazing around at home going to parties. On the other hand, you may feel that you want to do something entirely different from medicine to broaden your experience of the world. You might feel you would be more useful in a hospital or clinic only after you have almost completed your course. You will be encouraged to spend your elective period in the second or third clinical training years working in a Third World medical clinic, and you may decide therefore that that would be the best time when you will actually be more useful in a medical capacity.

Graduates

Most medical schools take a small number of graduates from other subjects to read medicine. Recently also, accelerated, fast-track, graduate courses that take only four years have been introduced mainly for those who have done science honours courses already. Given the competition for undergraduate places, however, unless there are truly exceptional circumstances, it may not be realistic to attempt to change to medicine unless you have got or expect to get at least a 2:1 in your first degree. Some universities also provide a few places for a premedical conversion course, often termed 1st MB, covering basic Chemistry, Biology, Maths and Physics for those who have done entirely Arts subjects until now. Often, however, it is only necessary to take A2-level Chemistry to qualify for consideration.

Even more so than with school leavers, interviewers of graduates will be concentrating on assessing the strength of your commitment to medicine. The obvious question is, if you are now so keen on studying medicine, why did you not apply from school? An honest answer would often be, 'I wasn't sure then, and anyway I didn't get good enough A levels.' Hence, you would have to be able to explain away the latter, and convince the panel that you are now utterly committed to medicine. (See also Chapter 6 on graduate entry medicine.)

Summary

■ Do spend a great deal of time investigating what medicine is really like at the coalface and thinking about how you would react to those conditions.

■ Talk to doctors, particularly junior ones, who can tell you what they find good and bad about their lives.

■ Be brutally honest in your examination of your character; do not confuse what you think you should be like with what, in your heart of hearts, you know you are really like.

■ If you still want to devote your life to medicine after all this introspection, try to get good GCSEs and do appropriate AS and A2 levels – at least Chemistry and perhaps an arts subject, aiming for at least AAB grades.

- Communicate in your personal statement your particular reasons for being enthusiastic about medicine, and demonstrate your intelligence, energy, wide interests and organization.
- Make sure that the teacher who writes your school report reinforces your claims.

Further reading

Visit the websites of the medical schools to which you are going to apply. British Medical Association website: www.bma.org.uk.

British Medical Association. *Medical Careers – A General Guide*. London: BMJ, 2001.

Hammond P, Moseley M. *Trust Me I'm a Doctor (An Insider's Guide to Getting the Most Out of the Health Service)*. London: Metro, 1999. (For a jaundiced and, I hope, outdated view.)

Richards P, Stockill S, Foster R *et al*. *Learning Medicine*. Cambridge: Cambridge University Press, 2006.

Your school's perspective

 3

Dr Simon Thorn, *Head of Biology, Radley College, Oxfordshire*

It might at first appear odd for a teacher to be giving advice on applying to medical school. I do, however, have a peculiar perspective on the process; I was a medical student myself before completing a BSc and PhD in Physiology. I abandoned research to become a biology teacher after an attack by animal rights activists.

Applicants' challenge

There is a need in this country for a supply of dedicated and able young medical students in order to maintain the standards of healthcare we expect. Due to the continually increasing number of applications for a limited number of places, it has been necessary for medical schools to make most selections on the basis of AS and A2-level grades. The level of offers made through UCAS has risen over the last 15 years from BCC to AAB. This deters less academic, but perfectly able, candidates. However, it encourages more academic students to consider medicine, rather than other degrees, on the basis of status.

How can this situation be alleviated? Medical schools cannot scout for talent – they can only consider those who apply. Places are offered on the basis of academic record, references, personal statement and, more often than not, interview. In addition, some medical schools have devised their own tests to provide further data as a basis for the selection of students. It is thus incumbent upon all secondary schools to encourage those of their sixth-formers who are best suited to medicine to apply, and to give them the best chance of fulfilling their potential.

What should a medic be like?

At a UCAS seminar for medical admissions tutors from all over Britain, teachers and tutors were asked to summarize the qualities looked for in MEDICS: see Figure 1. This rather banal mnemonic really encompasses a huge range of personal skills and attributes that medics should possess to varying degrees. As the training prepares medics for all careers within the

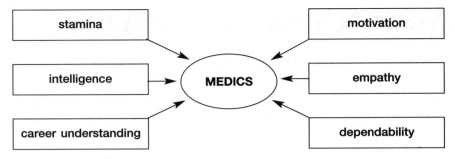

Figure 1 Qualities looked for in MEDICS

profession from pathology to psychiatry, a broad mix of students is essential. Nevertheless, the common elements might be exemplified thus:

- **motivation**: a commitment, drive and ambition to achieve goals
- **empathy**: a humane understanding of other people and willingness to put their comfort above your own
- **dependability**: an ability to consider problems and make decisions even under pressure, both as a team member and as a team leader
- **intelligence**: common sense and a quick grasp of concepts and factual details, with the ability to communicate effectively
- **career understanding**: an insight into the variety of skills, working conditions and stresses involved in practising medicine
- **stamina:** enough physical and emotional strength to cope with the course and the career.

Role of the secondary school

The selection and preparation process begins, to a certain extent, at school. Students who show an interest in studying medicine can be encouraged and helped to make decisions that are in their best interest, for example which A levels to choose, which undergraduate courses to select and which universities to apply to. I am not going to make any recommendations here except that students and teachers inform themselves. (See also Chapter 2 on entry requirements to medical school.)

I shall give some indication of the school's role in:

- acquiring medical knowledge
- gaining working experience

■ making the decision
■ UCAS advice
■ preparing for interview
■ getting the grades in A level.

Figure 2 summarizes the basic stages and steps involved in obtaining a place at medical school.

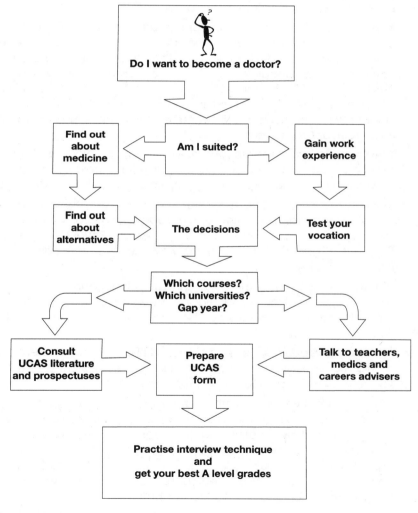

Figure 2 Schematic showing the decision process when applying to medical school

Where to get medical knowledge

There is a panoply of resources available. A school library or careers room should stock enough up-to-date material to keep students, teachers and parents informed. The main sources of information are listed below.

- **Books:** medical biography and history can enthrall, inspire or bore, in equal measures. Similarly, medical textbooks can fascinate or repel would-be medics.

- **Pamphlets:** UCAS and other publishers produce pamphlets with current advice and helpful information.

- **Journals:** *New Scientist* gives an appropriate overview of current issues and developments in science, including biomedical topics. Recent issues of the *British Medical Journal*, the *Lancet*, the *Journal of the Royal Society of Medicine*, etc., can be obtained from a helpful doctor. They all have editorial and news sections dealing with issues with which anyone interested in medicine should be familiar. The *Student BMJ* is particularly useful and readable, covering many of the issues relevant to students.

- **Newspapers:** the broadsheets have weekly medical and health features. Medical developments, scandals and policies are always newsworthy, and cuttings can easily be assembled into a scrapbook.

- **Internet:** the Internet can provide much of interest, but can also be a source of distraction. Choose your search keywords carefully. Surf the university websites and those of the various Royal Colleges (e.g. Surgeons, Physicians, etc.) and the Royal Society of Medicine and British Medical Association.

- **Videos:** television documentaries and medical soaps can provide extremely good stimulus material for group discussions on ethics. A valuable library of resources can be built up in a comparatively short time.

- **Prospectuses:** courses, towns and universities are all different. You should read about intake requirements, course structure and university facilities (such as accommodation and sports).

- **Clinical club:** There will be others at your school who will want to be doctors, vets, dentists, nurses, radiographers or physiotherapists. Much can be gained by meeting together regularly to discuss matters of concern such as ethical issues or to give talks on your own work experiences. The club will also give you a foretaste of the camaraderie that exists at medical schools, when you will be busy studying together while others are out partying.

How to gain work experience

Remember that before you can work in any healthcare setting, you must have been vaccinated against hepatitis B.

It can be quite daunting, and often difficult, arranging clinical observation or practical work experience. Some doctors and hospitals have been criticized in the past for having mere schoolchildren in potentially dangerous and highly sensitive clinical situations. Conversely, many doctors are keen to encourage the right person to join the profession.

Your school can help by developing a network of past pupils and parents who are medics. These doctors will have a personal interest in ensuring that you get the best possible learning experience. Many will also be happy to visit your school and give talks about their clinical work or research.

Similarly, with regular contact, your school can build up links with local practices and hospitals. These should not be restricted to giving help to prospective medical students. Schools can provide young people to help with voluntary work of all descriptions, from serving in a friend's shop to decorating children's wards at Christmas.

Do I want to be a doctor?

This is possibly the most difficult decision you need to make and one you must make yourself. There can be immense pressures on you to become a doctor: for example, there have always been doctors in your family; your parents always wanted you to be a doctor; the status of the job will be a step up the social ladder; your teachers say that, with your great academic potential, you owe it to yourself; and people keep saying what a great doctor you would make.

Remember, it is your decision and yours alone. To enable you to make that decision wisely, you must explore your vocation, as well as other academic alternatives.

Exploring your vocation involves testing your willingness and commitment to helping others even when it may be unpleasant for you. You may find voluntary work with the disabled or elderly extremely challenging but also rewarding. You should talk through your experiences with a medic as well, so that you can relate them to the career that might await you.

Exploring other academic alternatives involves finding out more about biomedical sciences. The research fields of physiology, biochemistry, anatomy, pharmacology and genetics, among many others, might provide the academic challenge you need while still satisfying your vocation to improve mankind's health and welfare.

UCAS

The process of applying through the Universities and Colleges Admissions System (UCAS) is, in some ways, different for you as a prospective medic. You have a very limited number of universities from which to choose – 32 in 2007 – and are restricted to applying to only four. You must also submit your application earlier than the general entry, 15th October in 2006. If you are thinking of taking a year out (called a gap year), consult your school's university liaison officer. If you want to apply for deferred entry, you will need to be a very strong candidate and to have made plans for your gap year by the time of your interview. You should keep in touch with your school if you want to apply after A level, and should ensure that you will be available for interview during your year out. (See also Chapter 5 on how to choose a medical school.)

Which university? What should guide your choices?

Although the quality and content of all courses must meet the criteria set down by the General Medical Council (GMC), their style and flavour are all very different. You should familiarize yourself with the distinction between the 'traditional' pre-clinical–clinical courses and the now more widespread 'integrated' courses. The degree of integration varies from school to school. You should also examine the balance between academic and clinical teaching: medical schools attached to hospitals incline towards clinical research, whereas university medical schools will have close associations with biomedical faculties. For example, Bristol is unique in having veterinary, medical and dental schools.

All medical schools prepare students for all branches of medicine, but it might be worth considering which hospitals are used in clinical rotations for medical students. Remember also that there is enormous competition for places, but the ratio of applicants per place varies. UCAS publish current statistics.

The details of your other choices are not revealed by UCAS to the universities. Your choice of two 'insurance' non-medical courses can be to the same university as any of your medical applications. If you do not succeed in getting into medical school first time, you can always apply to read medicine as a postgraduate after having completed a degree in another subject. Indeed, there are currently 11 four-year accelerated courses designed specifically for life-science graduates.

The city and university setting should also influence your choice: the course is long, so you want to be happy wherever you end up. After reading official and alternative prospectuses, leafing through tourist guides and talking to friends and family, you should visit those on your shortlist. The question you need to ask yourself is 'Do I feel at home?'

Your personal statement

There could be as many different pieces of advice on personal statements as there are medical admissions tutors – there is no right way. The most important feature is that it should be an honest account of your interest in and commitment to becoming a doctor. If you misrepresent yourself with regard to hobbies, books, places or people with which or whom you have had little real contact, you will be found out and everything you wrote that was true will be doubted.

Remember that the personal statement is just that. There is a temptation to allow parents and teachers to rewrite it to a point where the only original thought of yours on the page is 'I want to be a doctor'. Resist this! Your character must shine through. You should, nevertheless, write grammatically and spell correctly (these are basic skills that a doctor must have) and remember to follow the instructions on the UCAS website to the last detail.

You might find it helpful to structure your personal statement in sections covering:

- your reasons for studying medicine
- how you have found out about what it is like to be a doctor
- what you have gained from work experience
- your hobbies and interests within and outside school
- your outstanding qualities.

Your school's reference

The reference prepared by your school should be a fair assessment of your current academic and personal development. Each school will have its own format for preparing these references, but it is very important that the teacher(s) responsible for writing yours actually know(s) you. You should discuss with them your motives for becoming a doctor and the preparation you have done. They should also have a copy of your personal statement.

Your personal and academic strengths should be apparent and easily understood by the admissions tutors who will read the reference. One possible approach is to structure the reference thus:

- a general character reference
- individual subject references, including your predicted grades in boldface type
- an appraisal of your suitability for medicine as a course and a career.

How to prepare for interview

Most medical schools conduct interviews, but each has its own style and format. Some ask for examples of your work; some require you to complete a psychometric test; some set an admissions test or require you to take the BMAT (Bio-Medical Admissions Test; see www.bmat.org.uk) or UKCAT (UK Clinical Aptitude Test). To prepare yourself for these, you should:

- **Read the prospectus thoroughly.** You will look foolish if you appear ignorant of information to be found in the prospectus. Study the course structures and content. Find out about the accommodation and student facilities.

- **Take advantage of open days.** Your confidence and answers at an interview will reflect how well you feel at home in this relatively unfamiliar environment. Only by visiting the place and meeting the students will you be able to get a feel for it.

- **Practise your interview technique.** Your university interviews may be the first time you will experience the pressure of being questioned by unfamiliar people. The interview might be conducted by a panel or by just a couple of tutors. They will want to find out about you and your strengths. You should try to arrange practice interviews with your teachers and, if possible, a qualified doctor. The mock interviewers should have copies of your UCAS form and give you some feedback; this will help you to fill in some of the gaps in your knowledge and to conquer any nerves that might prevent your best qualities from shining through. You could even try recording interviews on video and criticizing your own weaknesses in presentation.

How to get the grade – No grades, no place

GCSEs

You should have a good portfolio of high grades at GCSE or Scottish Standard Grade. These should include English, Maths and separate or dual award sciences. Check prospectuses for individual university requirements. If you have qualifications other than GCSEs, you should contact each university admissions office for clarification.

A levels

Medical schools have all welcomed the opportunity given by Curriculum 2000 for an increase in breadth of study at A level, and most explicitly encourage you to take advantage of the system and take an AS (half an A level), or even A2 (a full A level), in an arts or humanities subject. To make yourself most widely acceptable to as many medical schools as possible, you should take Chemistry to A2 (although some will accept AS or even no Chemistry at all) and Biology or Biology (Human) to AS. Most medical schools have recognized that students coming in without Biology at A level have a lot of catching up to do. Some also suggest that Physics at AS is helpful. However, an exact combination is not prescribed; students are chosen on the basis of their personal qualities, not on a magic formula of subjects. In any case, you should be predicted at least grades AAB in A-level Chemistry (or Biology in the case of UEA and some other schools) and two other subjects (except General Studies). You may also have two A2 and two or more AS levels.

As the medical schools are continually developing their policies with respect to A levels, it is advisable to check their websites for the latest information on AS/A2 requirements, particularly with regard to retakes and the resitting of modules. Medical schools will not be prejudiced against applicants whose schools' policies are to 'cash in' or sit AS at the same time as A2 in Year 13 (upper sixth), rather than in Year 12 (lower sixth) in time to put results on the UCAS form. However, if you do have AS results, you should declare them on the UCAS form. Currently, certificated levels in Key Skills will not be stipulated. If you are taking IB (International Baccalaureate) or Scottish Highers, you should consult each university prospectus or website and the UCAS Handbook for specific requirements.

BMAT

Currently, Oxford, Cambridge, University College London (UCL) and Imperial College London (ICL) medical schools require applicants to sit a two-hour written test early in November (entries by the end of September). The BMAT (Bio-Medical Admissions Test) consists of multiple-choice, short-answer and short-essay questions covering aptitude, scientific knowledge, reasoning and communication skills. See www.bmat.org.uk for up-to-date information.

UKCAT

Since 2006, 23 medical schools have required candidates to sit the UK clinical aptitude test (UKCAT). This is a 90-minute test taken online at a Pearson VUE test centre before the end of September. The skills assessed include mental ability, problem-solving, logical reasoning, critical thinking and information management. See www.ukcat.ac.uk for up-to-date information and to register.

Study skills

Once you have received an offer, it is up to you to make the grade. There may be a temptation to relax, but you are barely halfway there. All universities make more offers than they have places, expecting that some of you will fail to reach their requirements. This means that under-scoring – even by one UCAS point – could cost you your place.

Ask your teachers how you are doing. If you are not on course for an A grade or you are not doing as well as you hoped, do not give up. Ask them what you need to do to improve. It will be a pleasure for them to see you work hard and achieve your ambition.

You may need to adjust your working and social habits. You might need to develop better reading and noting skills. You will certainly have to develop appropriate exam techniques. There are many revision and study guides available. Look at a few recommended ones and choose one that you like. You must be diligent about putting its advice into practice.

Summary

So, if you are serious about becoming a doctor:

- Find out about medicine.
- Gain work experience.
- Test your vocation.
- Seek advice on UCAS.
- Prepare for interviews. *
- Get the grades.

Further reading

Big Guide: The Official Universities and Colleges Entrance Guide, 2007. UCAS, 2006.
Medical Careers – A General Guide. BMA, 2001.
Progression to Medicine and Dentistry. UCAS, 2005.
Blundell A, Harrison R, Turney B. *The Essential Guide to Becoming a Doctor*. BMJ, 2004.
Burgess J, Girgis S, Hebert K. *The Insiders' Guide to UK Medical Schools 2005–6*. BMA, 2005.
Burnett J, Ruston J. *Getting into Medical School*. Trotman, 2006.
Butterworth J, Thwaites G. *Preparing for the BMAT: The Official Guide to the Biomedical Admission Test*. Heinemann, 2005.
Richards P. *A Student's Guide to Entry to Medicine*. UCAS, 1996.

Websites

'UCAS' at www.ucas.com.
'BBC – h2g2 – How to Get Into UK Medical School' at www.bbc.co.uk/dna/h2g2/A717527.

The interview

4

Professor John Stein, Medical Admissions Tutor, Magdalen College, University of Oxford

The majority of medical schools interview all applicants whom they feel have a reasonable chance of getting places. This means that about half of applicants are invited for interview, and most will get places. But, at present, Southampton, Belfast, Edinburgh and St Andrew's medical schools do not interview those who have not yet taken their A2 levels, i.e. pre-A-level candidates, at all.

There are two main aims of the interview:

■ to judge your enthusiasm, commitment and suitability for medicine
■ to assess your academic potential.

The latter is slightly less important for universities that concentrate less on the basic sciences behind medicine. Most of these are content with the evidence provided by your school report and your GCSE and AS/A2-level performance.

To assess your commitment, interviewers will definitely ask you in one way or another why you want to study medicine. There is no perfect answer to this question – but remember you are trying to sell yourself.

Do not be too modest. You should use the interview as an opportunity to explain your particular interests and enthusiasms in medicine, and what you have done to acquaint yourself with what medicine is really like through your work experience, voluntary service in a hospital, hospice, old people's home or clinic, hospital portering or service of other kinds.

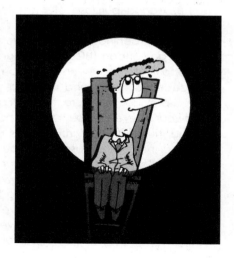

Your interviewers will also probably be interested in your views on current medical issues, such as the funding of the NHS, ensuring the quality of doctors' performance (which is now known as 'clinical governance'), euthanasia, or the pros and cons of the new genetics. So you need to have a little knowledge about these things and to have formed your own opinions on them. Again, there are no right answers: we are most interested in your appreciating both sides of the argument and how you make up your own mind.

Useful hints

■ Your reasoning will help your interviewers to judge how clearly you can think and how much you have bothered to find out about burning political and ethical issues in UK medicine.

■ They will also be trying to assess your enthusiasm, intelligence, energy and organization. So, in addition, they will probably ask you about your other interests – academic, cultural or sporting. Again, this is not because there is anything intrinsically better about being a county chess player, playing for your school 2nd XI at football or winning a ballroom dancing competition. They all show that you've got wider interests and that you can organize your time well enough to do well academically, yet also pursue your other interests to a high standard.

■ The public expect their doctors to be people they can admire and upon whom they can rely. Mainly, they trust your knowledge and experience of disease, but outward and visible symbols are important too. Therefore, even though your peers might think it uncool to wear a tie, dress smartly for your interview.

■ Do not be late, and prepare for the interview by, at the very least, having read the medical school's prospectus and knowing what it particularly has to offer.

■ The second purpose of the interview – and one that is especially important for medical schools that concentrate more on the basic sciences behind medicine, such as Oxford, Cambridge, University College London (UCL), Edinburgh and Imperial College London (ICL) – is for the interviewers to try to make a finer judgement about your academic ability and potential than GCSE and A-level predictions can provide. Therefore, they will probably ask you about some aspect of your A-level course that you have found particularly interesting. But ritual humiliation at interview is a thing of the past. Nowadays, we avoid trying to expose what you do not know by asking a stream of unrelated questions about your factual knowledge. Instead, most interviewers will try to find out what you are interested in, and then discuss that. What we are trying to do is to find out how you use the knowledge that you do have to support your arguments with evidence; how deeply you have delved into the subject to find out how it really ticks; how well you can think on your feet; and how clearly and logically you can express the results of your thought processes. Often you will be given a problem to solve there and then, or be taught something new to see how you cope with it.

■ Take things slowly, and do not be afraid to admit it if you think you have made a mistake. One of the most important things a doctor has to learn is to know when he or she is wrong.

Summary

■ At the interview, make sure that you have some knowledge about the special features of that medical school; be prepared to talk about current socio-medical and medico-political issues such as euthanasia or financing the health service; and, if you are applying for a course that emphasizes the basic sciences, be prepared to talk in some detail about why you are interested in them and how they relate to medicine.

■ Above all, communicate your enthusiasm, organization and energy.

How to choose a medical school

5

Emily Stobbs, *Medical Student, University of Nottingham*

So you have decided that becoming a doctor is the only thing you want to do. You are doing the right A levels, and you are pretty bright! However, where should you go to study for the next 4–6 years? This chapter will outline various factors you should take into consideration when choosing the four medical schools you are going to put down on your UCAS form.

Entry requirements

You have no doubt realized that you need to get top grades to do medicine, but there are a wide range of offers, which may sway your choice of medical school. Belfast, Edinburgh, Oxford, Cambridge and Dundee are currently the only schools that ask for 3As; the majority accept AAB and a few may accept ABB at A2 level. Although medicine has a reputation for being exclusive and only for the academically gifted, all medical schools have a policy on students who may have missed their intended grades. Therefore, do contact the medical school you are interested in to enquire about their resit policy. Also be aware that some medical schools ask for certain GCSE requirements – for example, Cambridge asks for a grade C or above in Physics, Maths and Biology.

BMAT (Bio-Medical Admissions Test)

This is an exam that a handful of medical schools require you to take. It is an hour in length and consists of both short-answer science questions and essay questions. If you are applying to Cambridge, Imperial College London (ICL), Manchester, Oxford or University College London (UCL), you must pass this exam in the November following sending your application to UCAS in October. (See also Chapter 2 on entry requirements to medical school.)

Interview versus personal statement

Your personal statement is the starting point for your application to medical school, so it **must** be outstanding (examples of your dedication/interest to study medicine – e.g. skills that you have that you will need as a doctor –

Table 1 Universities interviewing prospective medical students

Medical school	Interview?	Medical school	Interview?
Aberdeen	Yes	Leeds	Yes
Barts and the London	Yes	Leicester/Warwick	Yes
Birmingham	Yes	Liverpool	Yes
Bristol	Yes	Manchester	Yes
Brighton and Sussex	Yes	Newcastle	Yes
Cambridge	Yes	Nottingham	Yes
Cardiff	Yes	Oxford	Yes
Dundee	Yes	Peninsula	Yes
Durham	Yes	Queen's, Belfast	Not usually for
East Anglia	Yes		undergraduate
Edinburgh	Not usually		candidates
Glasgow	Yes	Sheffield	Yes
Kings, London	Yes	Southampton	Not usually
Hull/York	Yes	St Andrews	Yes
Imperial College London	Yes	Swansea	Yes
Keele	Yes	St George's, London	Yes
Lancaster (first cohort starting in 2007)	Yes	University College London	Yes

and relevant work experience). Some medical schools, including Belfast, Edinburgh, and Southampton, do not normally interview, and hence rely only on your personal statement. If your predicted grades are lower than you would like, perhaps an interview would be a good idea so that you can explain the reasons for your grades. Table 1 explains which universities interview prospective medical students.

Open days

Wherever possible, visit the medical school you are planning to apply to before you send off your UCAS form. There is only so much a prospectus can tell you, and it is hard to convey the atmosphere of the university through the written word. A prospectus will never say anything negative about the university, and to get a realistic prospective it would be advisable to go to an open day. It is also important to talk to current medical students at the schools you visit, to hear their impressions of where they are studying.

How will I be trained?

Traditional versus integrated and problem-based learning

Most schools now have an integrated approach to teaching medicine; that is, they have clinical contact in the first years alongside the basic science teaching, and then students start their clinical attachments sometime in the third or fourth year. When studying for a degree that will eventually lead you into a career working with people, many people feel it is important to get patient contact early on. However, if the concept of having to speak to patients so soon after you have begun your training fills you with dread, Oxford, Cambridge and St Andrews still offer the traditional medical degree, where there is a so-called 'pre-clinical/clinical divide'; that is, the first three years are academic, and the final years are clinical.

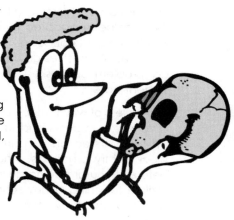

Table 2 Course structure at UK medical schools

Medical school	Course structure	Medical school	Course structure
Aberdeen	Integrated	Leicester/Warwick	Integrated, some PBL
Barts and the London	Integrated, some PBL	Liverpool	Integrated and PBL
Birmingham	Integrated	Manchester	Integrated and PBL
Bristol	Integrated		
Brighton and Sussex	Integrated	Newcastle	Integrated
Cambridge	Traditional (some clinical contact in first 3 years)	Nottingham	Integrated
		Oxford	Traditional (some clinical contact in first 3 years)
Cardiff	Integrated		
Dundee	Integrated		
Durham	Integrated	Peninsula	Integrated
East Anglia	Integrated and PBL	Queen's, Belfast	Integrated
		Sheffield	Integrated
Edinburgh	Integrated	Southampton	Integrated
Glasgow	Integrated	St Andrews	Traditional (transfer to Manchester Medical School for clinical years)
Kings, London	Integrated		
Hull/York	Integrated, some PBL		
Imperial College London	Integrated, some PBL	Swansea	Graduate entry only
Keele	Integrated and PBL	St George's, London	Integrated and PBL
Lancaster (first cohort starting in 2007)	Integrated and PBL	University College London	Integrated
Leeds	Integrated		

PBL: problem-based learning.

Problem-based learning (PBL) is a new approach to teaching medicine that has been adopted by a handful of medical schools (see Table 2). Problem-based courses are fully integrated, so they have clinical contact early on. PBL involves group work where students are usually given a clinical problem and asked to research it – hence learning is much more student-based.

Regardless of which medical school you choose, you can expect to have a variety of lectures and tutorials in small groups. Some medical schools still have dissection as part of their anatomy curriculum and some do biochemistry practicals. Once you start your clinical attachments (and before, if you are doing an integrated course), you will have ward-based clinical teaching. Many schools offer students the opportunity to undertake Special Study Modules (SSMs), where you can chose a particular area of interest to learn more about and to research into.

Table 2 outlines the course structure at each of the universities in the UK.

Location, location, location!

When deciding which of the 32 medical schools you want to apply to, you need to take into account a number of practical factors:

- **Cost** London is generally much more expensive to live in than most areas of the country, for accommodation, food, going out, etc.
- **Distance from family** Do you want to live at home to keep costs down? Would you rather be close enough so you can bring your washing home every weekend and be fed Sunday lunch on a regular basis? Or perhaps you would prefer complete freedom and want to go to university as far away from home as possible?
- **Campus site versus city site** Do you want to be at a medical school that is next to the rest of the university or a medical school that is separate from other faculties of the university?
- **Surroundings** Think about what you want on site or nearby. Do you want to be near the sea or the shops, the countryside or the capital?

Size of medical school

It may matter to you how many other students there will be in your cohort. Schools such as Cambridge are relatively small (with an intake of approximately 150) compared with, for example, Imperial College London, which has an intake of over 300 students per year.

Fancy a gap year?

If so, check that the medical schools you are applying to are happy for you to take a year out. Usually, if you take a gap year, medical schools want you to do something constructive with it, such as charitable work, work in a medically related field, etc.

Intercalation – the chance to get two degrees for (almost) the price of one!

At Imperial, the course is six years, because every student does a mandatory BSc (the final year of a conventional science degree) after the third year. Students can choose from 17 different BSc courses, and they complete taught courses on their chosen BSc and can also carry out research projects. At Nottingham, the course is the usual five years, but all students will also graduate with a BMedSci. They will cover the content of the BMedSci degree over the first three years while doing their regular medical training, and will have to write a dissertation in the third year to complete this degree.

Oxbridge students have to do a BA in their third year, completion of which allows students to apply for clinical school. Many medical schools offer the chance to take a year out of your medical studies to do a BSc. A typical requirement for this is that your exam results have to be in the top 10% for your year group. Glasgow offers either a one-year BSc (MedSci) or a two-year BSc after the third year, where you can study a BSc in more depth.

If you know what research you would be interested in doing for a BSc, find out which universities specialize in that field, and you can even mention in your personal statement that you are interested in that area of research.

Graduate Entry Medicine (GEM)

If you are a graduate with a 2:1 degree under your belt, you are eligible to apply for a fast-track four-year medical degree. Graduate entry is discussed in greater detail in Chapter 6.

Pre-medical courses

For those of you with good, non-science A levels, there is the opportunity to study for a six-year medical degree, with the first year in basic sciences. This course tends to have tougher entry requirements and spaces are limited. Schools that offer this are:

- Bristol
- Dundee
- Edinburgh
- Kings, London
- Manchester
- St George's, London
- Edinburgh
- Southampton.

Finance

As of September 2006, universities began charging up to £3000 per year for tuition fees – the so-called 'top-up fees'. This figure will increase each year slightly, with inflation. Not all universities will charge the maximum fees, so you need to check the individual university's prospectus or the UCAS website (www.ucas.ac.uk). However, unlike the old system, you will not have to pay your fees while you are at university. They only need to be paid back once you have left university and are earning over £15 000 per annum (which will be immediately after graduation for medics).

The student loan is still available for living expenses such as accommodation, food, travel, etc., but it is now called the Student Loan for Maintenance. It remains the same as previous years (increasing slightly per year due to inflation); for example, for 2006/2007, students living away from their parents' home and studying outside London are eligible for up to £4405 of a Student Loan for Maintenance. Seventy-five per cent of this figure is not income-assessed (i.e. everyone is eligible for this amount) and 25% is income-assessed (you may or may not be eligible, depending on your parents' income). This, like the tuition fees, is only repayable once you are earning over £15 000, and the only interest payable is linked to inflation. Basically, what all this means is that you will have less to pay while you are at university, but you will leave with more debt. For further information see Chapter 13 on student finance.

Summary

- You need to get top grades to get into medical school, but there is a wide range of offers.
- Although medicine has a reputation for being exclusive and only for the academically gifted, all medical schools have a policy on students who may have missed their intended grades.
- Wherever possible, visit the medical school you are planning to apply to before you send off your UCAS form.

▓ If you are applying to Cambridge, ICL, Manchester, Oxford or UCL, you must pass the BMAT.

▓ If you know what research you would be interested in doing for a BSc, find out which universities specialize in that area.

▓ Factors such as cost, distance from family, campus versus city site, and size of your medical cohort should all be considered when deciding which of the 32 medical schools you want to apply to.

Further reading

A *Guide to Financial Support for Higher Education Students in 2006/2007*. Student Finance Direct.

The Council of Heads of Medical Schools website, www.chms.ac.uk.

Graduate entry medicine

6

Dilshad Marikar, Graduate Medical Student, St George's Medical School, London

So you have got a degree and are ready for the challenge of studying medicine in only four years? Well, you have got a lot more choice than you used to: from five institutions offering such courses in 2002, there are now 14 medical schools offering graduate entry medical programmes.

This chapter will attempt to highlight some of the unique features of these programmes, and cast some light on the selection process and financial issues.

Is it right for me?

Perhaps the two most commonly cited features of graduate programmes compared with traditional undergraduate degrees are the 'advantage' of studying for four years rather than five or six, and the availability of a means-tested NHS bursary – which includes tuition fees – for years 2, 3 and 4. This is arguably the major reason why competition for places is so fierce.

Many graduate courses offer varying degrees of patient contact at an early stage, and teaching staff often described as enthusiastic and open to innovation. Obvious disadvantages include a more intense workload with less time to catch up if you fall behind, generally shorter holidays and less time for part-time work.

With regard to how these courses are structured and taught, it is not possible to generalize. Some may be run entirely separately from the five-year MBBS courses (as is the case at St George's at present), whereas on the graduate course at Guy's, King's and St Thomas' (GKT), students are taught separately only in their first year.

Many graduate entry courses use a problem- or case-based approach to drive the learning process, so it is essential to be sure that this is a method of learning that can work for you. For example, at St George's, the course is structured as themes – which are explored through problem-based learning (PBL). Students work in groups who are allocated their own 'base room' with a designated tutor. They are presented with weekly scenarios (patient case histories), which they explore with their tutor and from which learning objectives are generated; these objectives are satisfied through self-directed study, as well as activities organized for the week, which may include lectures, clinical skills sessions, hospital visits and seminars. At the end of the week, students consult experts in the area of medicine they are studying at an 'expert forum'. At the start of the following week, the previous week's case is wrapped up, with all the learning objectives (hopefully) resolved. Topics are revisited through many cases. So what does this achieve? According to the prospectus:

> By covering the knowledge base needed to understand different aspects of the problem, you will gradually acquire all the knowledge needed for the practice of medicine.

So did that pen portrait of problem-based learning whet your appetite or fill you with horror? To reiterate, course structures will vary, so read the prospectuses carefully. Go to open days if you possibly can. The open days I have been on have included a demonstration of the learning process, and gave a good opportunity to talk to current students.

Getting in

Around half of the graduate programmes will accept candidates with degrees from any discipline. The others require a first degree in science. A number make use of entrance exams as part of the selection criteria – which we will get onto shortly. Table 1 (adapted with permission from the 'Mature FAQ' – see Further reading) gives a list of the requirements in 2007.

Entrance exams

Ten graduate entry medical courses require sitting of entrance exams as part of your application, with intimidating acronyms: GAMSAT, BMAT, UKCAT and MSAT.

GAMSAT (Graduate Medical School Admissions Test)

GAMSAT is required for applications to St George's, Nottingham and Swansea for candidates with degrees from any discipline (the five-year MBBS at Peninsula also accepts GAMSAT). St George's and Nottingham use it as a selection criterion for interview, whereas at Swansea it is part of the scoring system after interviews have taken place – so it has no bearing on the chances of being called up for interview.

Table 1 Requirements for graduate entry

University	No. of places	Degree restrictions	Other qualifications	Entrance exam
Birmingham	40	Life science 2:1 (mostly 1sts)	A-level chemistry at grade 'C' or better	None
Bristol	19	Life/medical science 2:1	'Applicants must have covered a substantial component of cell biology and mammalian physiology in their previous degree'	None
Cambridge	20	'Good degree in any discipline'	Complex – consult admissions website	BMAT
Guy's, King's and St Thomas'	24	2:1 arts or science	—	MSAT
Leicester	64	2:1 health science	—	UKCAT
Liverpool	32	2:1 in biological/healthcare	Minimum BBB at A level including Biology and Chemistry	None
Newcastle	25	2:1 (almost all 1sts)	Any within last 2–3 years	None currently
Nottingham*	91	2:2	—	GAMSAT
Oxford	30	Life science/chemistry 'usually 2:1 or better'	Two science A levels or equivalent; if degree is Chemistry, must have GCSE/O-level Biology or better	UKCAT
Queen Mary	40	2:1 in science or health-related subject	—	MSAT
Southampton	40	2:1	GCSE passes in English, Maths and Science; AS Chemistry and Biology or A2 Chemistry	None
St George's*	70	2:2	—	GAMSAT
Swansea	70	2:1	Chemistry or Biology at AS/A/degree level	GAMSAT (only used as part of their scoring system)
Warwick	164	2:1 biological sciences (or 2:2 biological sciences with subsequent doctorate)	A levels/GCSEs not considered	MSAT

*Candidates who have applied for both Nottingham and St George's will be interviewed once, as both institutions share the interview process but differ on the interview score required to get an offer; applicants rejected by St George's have been known to be offered a place at Nottingham.

GAMSAT is administered by UCAS, and costs £176 (the price includes a small packed lunch). It takes place in September and consists of three papers with breaks in between. The three papers are:

▓ **Section I:** Reasoning in the Humanities and Social Sciences (multiple-choice) – 100 minutes

▓ **Section II:** Written Communication (two 30-minute essays) – 1 hour

▓ **Section III:** Reasoning in Biological and Physical Sciences – Biology 40%, Chemistry 40%, Physics 20% (multiple-choice) – 170 minutes.

The overall mark is calculated so that a strong showing in Sections I and II can compensate for a relatively poor showing in Section III and vice versa. Interviews are offered to everyone who achieves the cut-off mark decided. In 2006, the cut-off score for St George's and Nottingham was 62.

At five and a half hours long, GAMSAT has been described as an unpleasant endurance test (there are breaks between papers, of course). There are a number of practice tests and even courses available to prepare for GAMSAT, but probably the first and best investment you can make in terms of preparing for the exam is to purchase the official sample and practice papers – see the links at the end of this section.

A fact sheet prepared by previous applicants suggests that A-Level knowledge of Biology and Chemistry can be sufficient for Section III; be warned, though, that historically there have been a significant number of questions on organic chemistry. Remember that you need to achieve at least the minimum required marks in all three sections, so don't neglect your comprehension and essay writing skills at the expense of science!

Finally, it is worth noting that a GAMSAT score is valid for two years, so if you get a good mark and wish to apply for the following year, you need not necessarily sit the test again.

BMAT (Bio-Medical Admissions Test)

BMAT is used by the Cambridge graduate-entry course and a number of five-year courses. It is a two-hour, pen-and-paper test consisting of three sections:

▓ **Section 1:** Aptitude and Skills (60 minutes – 35 multiple-choice or short-answer questions)

▓ **Section 2:** Scientific Knowledge and Applications (30 minutes – 27 multiple-choice or short-answer questions)

▓ **Section 3:** Writing Task (30 minutes – one from a choice of three short-essay questions).

The science section assesses basic science knowledge (at the level of GCSE Double Science and Maths). Although a far shorter exam than

GAMSAT, the science section is considered to be quite challenging due to time pressure and the nature of the questions. A calculator is not allowed in the exam, so good arithmetic skills help! Sample questions are available on the BMAT website.

MSAT (Medical Schools Admissions Test)

MSAT is used by GKT, Queen Mary's and Warwick graduate entry courses. It has a somewhat similar format to GAMSAT, but is somewhat different in content. It does not have a science paper. The exam consists of three sections:

- **Part I:** Critical Reasoning/Problem Solving (multiple-choice) – 65 minutes
- **Part II:** Interpersonal Understanding (multiple-choice) – 55 minutes
- **Part III:** Written Communication (two 30-minute essays) – 60 minutes.

UKCAT (UK Clinical Aptitude Test)

The UK Clinical Aptitude Test (UKCAT) is a new entrance test developed by a consortium of universities. Applicants to graduate-entry courses at Leicester and Oxford are required to sit it. Unlike the other tests, UKCAT is computer-based.

From the information currently available, it appears that UKCAT does not test scientific knowledge; rather, it has questions on verbal, numerical and abstract reasoning, as well as problem-solving questions. Also, the exam will not necessarily have a pass mark, but results will be used by each medical school as part of the overall assessment of the candidate.

Can I get in with a 2:2?

Without a doubt, getting a medical school to consider your application with a 2:2 degree (and no postgraduate degree) is difficult. Of the graduate-entry courses, the only two institutions that will consider you equally with those with higher degree classes are St George's and Nottingham – if you are willing to sit the GAMSAT exam and achieve the cut-off mark (see below). GKT will accept a lower second-class honours degree with a postgraduate degree, while Warwick requires a doctorate. As ever, before you put down an institution on UCAS, consult admissions so as to know whether you have a realistic chance of being considered.

Interviews

On applying, you may well be faced with a structured interview, and, depending on the medical school, interviewers may or may not have access to your personal statement and academic details. Expect questions aimed to cast light on your motivation, ability to deal with stress, integrity, character and empathy! Interviews at St George's and Nottingham last for 40 minutes, so you will need to be able to articulate on lessons learnt from your work (and life) experience.

Funding

As a graduate, your local education authority is unlikely to approve support for tuition fees; so unless you did not receive public funding for your first degree, tuition fees for the first year need to be paid by you.

Thankfully, graduates are still eligible for student loans. At the time of writing, if you live outside London, you could receive a student loan of up to £4405 a year (£6170 if based in London, £3415 if you are living with your parents). Of this loan entitlement, you are guaranteed at least 75%, which is the non-income-assessed portion. Your eligibility for the remaining 25% is dependent upon your household income. In addition, as graduate courses generally have longer terms than the five-year courses, a supplementary loan is available for each week above the standard 30 weeks of term time. In the years that students are entitled to NHS bursaries (i.e. from the second year onwards), you will be entitled to a reduced-rate maintenance loan (around 50%).

The Department for Education and Skills (DfES) provides additional support for students with children or adult dependents, as well as students with disabilities. Details are available from the DfES website: www.dfes.gov.uk/studentsupport/students/index.shtml.

The NHS bursary

English and Welsh students on graduate-entry courses are eligible for the NHS bursary from years two to four. Scottish students are currently not eligible. The bursary consists of a main allowance to cover day-to-day living costs. This amounts to £2309 a year for those living outside London (£2837 if you are based in London, £1889 if you are living with your parents). Graduate entry students also receive a weekly rate fro each extra teaching week above 30 weeks and 3 days. On top of this, significant additional allowances are available (examples include a dependants' allowance, tuition contributions, placement costs and disabled students' allowance). The bursary is means-tested; however, any casual earnings you make as a full-time student are disregarded up to £7500.

Detailed information on the NHS bursary is available in the booklet *Financial Help for Health Care Students*, available at www.nhspa.gov.uk/sgu/Forms/Booklets/students_financial_help.pdf.

Summary

▨ The competition for graduate entry medicine places is fierce and the workload is challenging.

▨ You should expect a well-organized, challenging and enjoyable course.

▨ Make sure you do your own 'homework' in knowing about entry requirements for the medical school of your choice.

▨ Good luck on getting your place!

Further reading

The Mature FAQ – a regularly updated and comprehensive document that provides advice for the 'chronologically challenged' on getting into medical school.

www.geocities.com/alexism1974/maturefaq.htm

Medschool online maintains a section on graduate entry medical programmes, including information on applications per place offered.

www.medschoolsonline.co.uk/.

Further information on GAMSAT

UCAS GAMSAT page: www.ucas.com/tests/gamsat.html

GAMSAT information booklet:
www.acer.edu.au/tests/university/gamsatuk/intro.html

Med school guide GAMSAT forum: www.medschoolguide.co.uk.

Further information on BMAT

www.bmat.org.uk/index.html.

UKCAT website

www.ukcat.ac.uk/

Student finance

Andrew Pearson, *Former Finance Chair, BMA Medical Students Committee*
Kirsty Lloyd, *Former Chair, BMA Medical Students Committee*

A key issue in many minds when considering entering medicine is finance. This chapter should help you to become a little clearer on how finances work for medical students.

How will I pay my way through medical school?

The funding you will receive through medical school will depend upon the following:

- which UK country you live in before you enter higher education
- whether you have done a degree before
- your parental or spousal income (depending on age/circumstances).

It is important to carefully investigate what government financial support you will be eligible for, as many 'headline' figures are the maximum available, and subject to an individual's circumstances. A useful first place to start would be the Royal Medical Benevolent Fund's Finance for Medical Students Website and the relevant government website for the area where you have lived for at least three years (not including university, if you have a first degree) – known as the place you are 'domiciled' in. Some medical students are entitled to receive grants or bursaries; these don't need to be paid back. It is worth checking carefully to see if you are eligible. However, the most significant part of most medical student's income will be the student loan.

The student loan

There are two types of student loan:

- a 'free loan' – paid straight to your university to cover fees
- a 'maintenance loan' – paid directly to the student to live on.

Interest is paid on the student loan at the rate of inflation; in real terms, this means you will pay back what you borrowed. Once you graduate, the student loan repayments are taken out of your earnings along with tax, and only on earnings of greater than £15 000. Therefore, while you will take many years to pay off a student loan, it is still considered as the best form of debt to be in. As some of the student loan is means-tested, many medical students do not receive the full student loan. There are additional means of obtaining enough money to live on.

Bank loans

Most high-street banks offer overdrafts to students, and some offer additional commercial loans that are available to medical students later on in the course. These will need to be paid back quicker than student loans, and the bank loans charge a commercial rate of interest. It is worth shopping around to see what would suit you best, and be prepared to move all your banking to the bank that offers you a loan. It is worth remembering that banks are not obliged to lend to everyone, and will want to see that you have had an address in the UK for a number of years. A bad credit history may not help – so be sure you pay those bills off on time!

The bank of Mum and Dad

Many students will receive some financial support from their family. In fact, depending on your family circumstances, the government will expect them to provide financial support. This is calculated via 'means testing': your parents/spouse/partner will be required to provide detailed financial information about their earnings and the family outgoings, and the government then calculates how much money you can borrow from a student loan and how much your family is expected to pay to you. There are circumstances in which a student is considered to be 'independent' of their parents – and the government's view on this and your own view may be very different. It is important to check what the regulations are and talk it over with your family. The current criteria to be considered 'independent' of your parents may change; however, at present the parents of most students under 25 are means-tested. Some students find that on paper their families are required to contribute but in the real world are not able to. It is known that around one in eight of those medical students who have their entitlement reduced due to their parents' income do not receive the financial support from their parents that the government has calculated.[1]

Students in this position still study medicine – it means that they become more resourceful and have to investigate other financial options, such as bank loans.

Other sources of funding

Money that doesn't increase your debt is also available. There are a number of charitable trust grants available to medical students, for which you will have to fill in an application form and meet specific requirements regarding eligibility. Many charities have one annual deadline; others have ongoing submission dates. Research is the key to accessing this type of funding – you don't want to spend several days completing an application only to find out that you have to be a student who can do handstands while whistling to apply! Money given to students from charities often has certain conditions applied: for example, the money can only be used for an elective, or only for living costs. You must also be prepared to provide detailed personal financial information and keep good records of your spending. Often not many people apply for these grants, so it is certainly worth getting a list of these charitable trusts and writing to them when you are at medical school.

There are also university grants provided by many universities to students from low-income families. These are available to some students doing medicine as a first degree in certain years and depend largely on your parents' income (unless you qualify as 'independent' of your parents). They vary enormously (by thousands of pounds per year) between universities. If this is to be a factor in your choice of medical school, then it is important that you check very, very carefully that you are actually eligible for the relevant grant and how much.

Part-time jobs

Many medical students, particularly in the early part of their courses, have a part-time job. Working part-time has many benefits in addition to the financial reward. It can develop your CV and your communication skills, and introduce you to a wide variety of new people outside your course. For some students, part-time work will be the only way that they can get through medical school; for others, it is a decision taken to limit the amount of debt they are in. It is important to balance how much employment you undertake and how much time you devote to your studies, remembering that the cost of retaking a year – or, even worse, getting thrown out of medical school – will be far higher than the earnings from your job. Therefore the type of work, flexibility of hours and level of pay are important to consider. Some medical students undertake work that will help them in the future (such as auxiliary nursing), while others welcome the opportunity to get out of the medical setting and do something completely different. The advantages of working within hospitals are numerous: the shifts are flexible, hospital trusts are used to medical students, and it can help with your studies. Taking advantage of the longer summer holidays (if you have them) and working to save for the next academic year is also an important income source for many students.

Budgeting

Planning your time and your finances is important so as not to miss out completely on the numerous social and recreational activities that university life presents. Budgeting is an important part of living away from home and being at university. If you budget carefully, you will find that limited finances can go a very long way indeed. It is about achieving a balance in your life between studying, paid work, and going out and making the most of the opportunities that university has to offer. Ask someone who has already left home how they calculate their budget. An online budget planner can be found on many bank websites. You may already know if you are 'good' or 'bad' with money. If you are the latter, then budgeting will save you anxious moments at the end of term when you are not sure how you will pay your rent or buy food for the month before the next loan instalment arrives.

Why do medical students get into more debt than other students?

Medicine is a longer course and has longer terms, and therefore shorter holidays in which to earn money. The workload of the course can make it difficult to undertake employment during term time. Toward the end of the course, the time commitment increases, as you are often expected to be working at least 35 hours a week in hospital and most students are preparing for final examinations. There are also additional costs to a medical degree: equipment costs, travel to clinical placements, the 'elective' and the costs of having appropriate ward clothes.

Top tips for keeping costs down

- Buy only essential equipment, such as a good stethoscope.
- Apply early for your elective.
- Seek financial support from charities.
- Share lifts with other students to placements.
- Use the library. Library facilities vary: some medical schools will have superb facilities with 24-hour access and numerous copies of core textbooks, while other schools will have poorer facilities with restricted opening hours, and therefore you may need to purchase more books.

Table 1 Average expenditure by medical students[1]	
Monthly costs	
Travel to lectures	£41
Travel to attachments	£48
Food (at home and meals out)	£105
Entertainment	£84
Personal items	£46
Household items/running costs	£45
Yearly costs	
Textbooks/course materials	£154
Medical equipment	£62
Travel home	£172

If you like to study in a library environment, then you may need to buy fewer books at medical school. A breakdown of national 2004–2005 costs is presented in Table 1.

- Once you are convinced that a certain book suits your needs, you might like to buy it, but so often students buy what is on a reading list to find that the style of the writing is not for them.
- Sharing books with housemates is another way to get a wider personal library.

How much debt will I get into?

The amount of debt medical students get into is hugely variable. It depends on where they study, the funding they are eligible for, their course costs and whether they receive support from their family. Thus it is important to remember this when looking at 'average' levels of debt. In 2005, the average debt medical students were graduating in was around £21 000;[1] these students did not pay 'top-up fees', so it is likely that this figure will be significantly higher in the future.

Will my choice of medical school affect how much debt I get into?

While there are some costs that all medical students will incur, the amounts vary from medical school to medical school. The distance travelled to clinical attachments varies from school to school. Occasionally, medical schools will provide some funding or transport, and some medical students will receive limited assistance from their local education authority to cover this. The local costs of living are an important consideration when working on your budget – in particular the cost of

Table 2 Average monthly expenditure on accommodation by medical students by region of study[1]

Region	Cost (£)
London	388
Rest of England	272
Scotland	282
Wales	219
Northern Ireland	193

accommodation (Table 2). This can vary across the country. The obvious example is London, where generally the cost of living is significantly higher than in the rest of the UK, particularly for accommodation.[2]

What if my situation is more complicated?

The rules around eligibility for funding have become enormously complicated recently for a minority of students. If you have moved between the home nations (even a long time ago), have already done a degree, have spent time abroad recently, or are from elsewhere in Europe, the situation is more complex and beyond the scope of this book. If you are in this situation, then contact one of the organizations listed in Further reading, remembering that those you speak to will not necessarily deal with cases like yours regularly. Be patient but persistent in finding out your eligibility.

What if it all goes wrong and I get into financial difficulty?

Managing finances for the first time can be difficult, and not everyone gets it right. Financial hardship is a reality for many students, and the complicated systems of support can be hard to navigate. Seek advice and support at the earliest opportunity. Every university has a welfare and support officer. These are staff employed by the university to be experts in student finance. They will help you with financial planning, and will advise you on whether you have accessed all the money you are entitled to. There is also financial support available to students in difficulty, whether it is because you cannot work due to illness, or have an unexpected electricity bill or have simply run out of money. The government gives each university extra money to help students facing financial hardship; this is given as a grant that you do not have to pay back. Banks charge fees for going overdrawn without authorization, and also for bounced cheques or returned direct debits. It is vital to let the bank know if you are having trouble keeping within your limits; they may be able to waive charges while you sort things out. Seek advice as soon as you realize that there may be problems. Financial difficulties have far-reaching effects, and it is not unusual for anxiety in this area to affect your studies.

Summary

- The financial arrangements for medical students are far from ideal, leaving most with high levels of debt upon graduation. The numerous anomalies in the funding systems leave medical students in difficult situations.

- There are various student groups who lobby for changes to the system.

- Although managing your finances is a vital part of everyday life, and doing this with little or no real income can be incredibly difficult, very few medical students will regret the decision to study medicine for financial reasons.

- Training to become a doctor is a privilege that exposes you to different experiences every day, and, whatever their financial situation, most medical students will still be very glad they came to medical school – if you don't believe this, just ask them!

References

1. *Medical Student Finance Survey 2004–2005*. Health, Policy and Economic Research Unit, BMA.
2. Corps L, Urmston I. *The Insiders' Guide to Medical Schools (The Alternative Prospectus) 1999*. London: BMJ Publishing, 1999.

Further reading

English-domiciled students studying in the UK:
studentfinance.direct.gov.uk/index.htm

Northern Irish-domiciled students studying in the UK:
www.delni.gov.uk/index.cfm/area/information/page/StudentFinance

Scottish-domiciled students studying in UK and non-UK EU students* studying in Scotland: www.saas.gov.uk/

Welsh-domiciled students studying in the UK:
www.studentfinancewales.co.uk/

*'EU students' here means students who are EU citizens and are domiciled outside the UK but within the EEA or Switzerland.

Non-UK EU students* studying in England and Wales:
www.dfes.gov.uk/studentsupport/eustudents/index.shtml

International students (non-EU students*): www.dfes.gov.uk/international-students/

NHS tuition fee and grant page for English-domiciled students studying in the UK, and non-UK EU-domiciled students studying in England, in years 2, 3 and 4 of the accelerated programme or 5 and 6 of the normal programme: www.nhsstudentgrants.co.uk/

*'EU students' here means students who are EU citizens and are domiciled outside the UK but within the EEA or Switzerland.

The medical student years and how to survive them

8

Dr Faheem Shakur, F1 Houseman, General Medicine, The Royal Preston Hospital, Preston, Lancashire
Stuart Laverack, Final-year Medical Student, University of Sheffield

In recent years, studying medicine has changed, and so too has university life in general. There are now new methods of teaching, but also larger financial burdens on students. Having said this, medicine continues to be a very worthwhile and popular degree to study.

This chapter highlights the aspects pertinent to the successful completion of your medical school years.

The pre-clinical years

British medical courses are generally five or six years long (the extra year usually culminating in the award of a BMedSci/BSc or BA in Oxford or Cambridge). These are optional degrees that give the opportunity to do an extra amount of personal research into a chosen specialty.

There are two types of course on offer:

- PBL (problem-based learning)
- systems- or subject-based learning.

PBL is a way of learning that is completely different from what most of you are used to, and is becoming increasing popular at university. PBL involves small-group work around a particular clinical scenario, working together to teach yourselves the knowledge needed. While you are supervised, the emphasis is on finding the information for yourself. The good points of PBL are that it allows you to manage your workload more freely and that, if done correctly, it can make you very good at researching. However, the group needs to work together to get the work done and make the sessions interactive.

In comparison, the traditional systems/subject-based courses involve predominantly dissection and lectures, with some laboratory work. Normally, this section of the course is two to three years long. Some universities adopt a systems approach, where you work through each part of the body step by step, while others prefer a subject approach, with each discipline such as physiology or biochemistry being covered in turn.

Anatomy dissections (available in PBL and didactic teaching) are nothing like you expect and not at all as they are portrayed in the media. Either you will be given a whole cadaver to work on or prosections will be used. A demonstrator will normally supervise small groups and facilitate your learning. Over the weeks and months, you will slowly reveal just what the human body is made of. Many students start with the idea that dissection can be quite gruesome, but the vast majority of students view it as a highly effective learning tool.

A lecture can be either the most fascinating hour you can spend at university or the most mind-numbingly boring hour of your life. This experience is dependent on the style of the lecturer. Some can be interactive when a handout is worked through, while others can use the more archaic route of reading slides from a PowerPoint presentation. The aim of the lecture is to clarify points you will be reading about in textbooks.

There is also time in the laboratories studying subjects from histology to biochemistry. This time is often very interactive, bringing topics from a textbook to life. These sessions definitely cement ideas into your mind much better than hours spent in the library reading about them – seeing is believing.

The clinical years

By far the best part of the course is when one has the opportunity to talk to patients. Increasingly, clinical placements are starting earlier on in the degree, compared with the past. The clinical years are a bewildering yet inspirational, formative part of the course. They help to establish patient rapport, underscore the duties of a doctor and provide medical students with key practical skills. They also provide the ideal chance to lay the foundations for good history-taking and examination skills as required from a junior house officer right up to consultant level. There is much emphasis on professional behaviour – now so more than ever in the post-Shipman era.

The clinical years are integral to the development of good clinical skills for future doctors. However, the time spent doing your clinicals varies greatly. The majority is spent in hospitals, although plenty of time is given to working in general practice. There are ward rounds and clinical meetings to attend. Time is spent observing and assisting in operations, and there are many opportunities for history-taking and developing thorough clinical examination techniques. You are able to become part of the team and thereby understand how clinical decisions are made.

The different major specialties are studied in the clinical years, including psychiatry, obstetrics and gynaecology, and paediatrics. These can be very rewarding attachments, with equally demanding examinations following them.

Clinical attachments

Clinical attachments take place at university and peripheral hospitals. As a general rule, the university hospitals offer specialties and treatments not seen in smaller hospitals. If you are placed in a peripheral hospital, try to make the most of it, whether by gaining extra practical experience in a setting where there are fewer medical students per patient or by building contacts in the medical world.

During the clinical course, students have the opportunity to undertake special study modules to allow them to study further aspects of the course that are of particular interest to them. The GMC (General Medical Council) recommends that, in addition to the core curriculum covering the essential components of the MBChB degree, 25–33% of the course be allocated to the Student Selected Component Programme (SSC). Audit and other forms of research are catered for too. Audits look at current practice, in particular the clinical environment, and then try to provide suggestions for further improvement. Research can be fitted either alongside concurrent clinical attachments or as a separate entity in itself consisting of a year out and the achievement of a BMedSci/BSc.

Some medical schools provide a research year as standard, whereas in other universities this is optional or for those who do well in examinations. The research year provides an opportunity to delve deeper into a specific part of medicine, and may even lead into a career in academic medicine. (See also Chapter 15 on academic medicine.)

Examinations

Exams are a continual part of any medical professional's career, even after graduating from medical school. To become members of postgraduate medical institutions such as the Royal College of Physicians or the Royal College of Surgeons, one has to take quite a few exams. As you would expect, exams are therefore quite stressful and a big step up from what you have done before at school. The format of each exam varies with the course. For example, for subjects such as anatomy and histology, there is the *spotter exam*. This type of exam requires the candidate to identify specimens and answer questions related to the function of that particular specimen.

EMQs (extended matching questions), MCQs (multiple-choice questions) and essay papers are used throughout the course, either at the end of a particular module or at the end of the year.

- **EMQs** are questions for which the candidate is given a list of possible answers for each individual question. There is only one correct answer from the list of possible answers. Your job is simple: just select the correct one.

- **MCQs** are questions for which one has to answer true/false to the stated question. While this type of examination may sound simple, it is far from it, with the questions or answers being particularly ambiguous at times. Hence, always READ THE QUESTION.

- **Essay** papers seek greater depth of knowledge in a particular topic in a prose format.

- **Vivas** are oral exams, in which candidates are questioned by a group of examiners on a topic, and, rather than writing the answer, one has to explain the answer. Such exams are used in pass/fail or distinction scenarios.

During clinical attachments, there will be assessments. Assessments in a clinical setting prove that patients are not the same as described in textbooks, and that although a disease is said to have five symptoms, not every patient will show them. The clinical exam of choice in most medical schools and used particularly for medical finals is the OSCE (Objective Structured Clinical Examination). This is where an examiner will observe you with a patient (either simulated or real), testing your clinical examination or history-taking skills. Usually, only 5–10 minutes is allowed for this, thus adding to the pressure. Keeping one's cool in such an exam is of great importance, especially when it seems you are being asked a lot of questions pertaining to your particular case.

Hints for exams

- Be prepared and so start revising early.
- Remember everyone is in the same situation as yourself.
- Get plenty of rest the night before the exam.
- Try to keep exams in perspective; trying to revise when overstressed is far from ideal.

The elective

The elective is seen by many as the highlight of the medical course, and is undertaken at all the medical schools. It usually involves a clinical attachment ranging in length from one to three months. The clinical attachment can be done anywhere in the world, and many students use this opportunity to explore a number of exotic locations.

The elective is seen by some as a glorified holiday – it is, however, whatever you make of it. The opportunities are endless, given enough time and planning. You could be working in the real ER in Chicago or be helping with relief medicine in one of the countries affected by the tsunami. You could be the only medic available to a region of the developing world or seeing new treatments/technologies in wealthy countries. Also, being in an exotic location means that you will have to try new and exciting things, like skydiving in Fiji or bungee jumping in New Zealand.

Nevertheless, the elective is something that often is recounted after graduation as a highlight of medical school! The reason for this is that it is generally seen as a time when students are able to relax slightly and experience new cultures and make new friends across the world.

Life outside medicine – play hard, work hard

Upon starting medical school, there are a whole range of medical societies that students can join. A couple of the most popular ones are the RSM (Royal Society of Medicine) and BMA (British Medical Association). They have very attractive packages for medical students and cater for many medical needs throughout medical school. In addition to that, medics have the luxury of joining not only the relevant medics sport teams but also general university sport teams! People can also give up their free time for altruistic things such as volunteering, and this also looks brilliant on the CV as well as being generally satisfying for the soul.

As a medic, you will need to be able to convey your message to the wider public, so working with people or playing sports or any hobby that gives you access to people of all ages and ethnic groups is a brilliant idea. It will also improve your confidence, which is also useful in the adrenaline-charged situations you may find yourself in the future.

Remember there is a whole world outside medicine. Get involved in activities outside medicine, as in later years you will come to find support in a world away from the hospital. At university, there is so much available you will not be stuck for choice.

Finance

From September 2006, universities have been able to charge tuition fees of £3000 per year. Not all students will be subject to these tuition fees, as they depend on your financial situation. As with other degrees, student loans for maintenance are available to help with living costs. However, during the last one or two clinical years of your course, the NHS does provide a bursary to cover your university tuition fees.

Approximately one-quarter of medical students have a job during term time, and over half work during the holidays as well. Sometimes these jobs are medically linked, such as auxiliary nursing, working in a nursing home, typing reports in a GP practice or phlebotomy, or they may be completely unrelated to medicine.

The National Union of Students estimates that students spend nearly £100 a month on socializing and have average rents of between £40 to £100 per week, not to mention textbooks and other bills. Coming to university can be expensive, especially since medical courses are longer than most other degree courses. However, do not let your financial situation put you off applying – help is available to those in need, either before you start your degree or during it if your circumstances should change. (See also the Chapter 7 on student finance).

Life after university – becoming a doctor

With recent changes to the application process for applying to work as a doctor, university provides good opportunities to expand your CV. Make sure you try some volunteer work or get involved in something in your local community. There are also medical and surgical societies that you can join. Do not leave it until your final year to undertake such activities. Not only will you not have so much to put on your CV, but also you will have missed out on numerous exciting opportunities. After the hard work you have put in at medical school, enjoy the fruits of your labour and apply that knowledge on your future patients. (See also Chapter 10 on the foundation years).

Summary

- Make sure to make the most of your vacation time, as after the first year has ended this generally is the only long holiday you will have.
- You should have coping mechanisms for stress – playing sports, etc. There will be days when you will return from placement stressed, and while for some of you the way to relieve this stress may be to go for a drink with your mates, perhaps you should consider something else.

- Group study is often helpful, in particular for OSCEs (Objective Structured Clinical Examinations).
- Do not underestimate the stresses of living at university and simply coping as an adult at university.
- Learn to work with your friends: not only is this a good way to spread the workload and stress, it is also good practice for your years ahead as a doctor working within a medical team.
- Do not be shy in approaching your seniors or tutors for support during the course. Most of your predecessors are all too happy to make you aware of the pitfalls in the course.

Links

- www.gpnotebook.co.uk
- www.rsm.ac.uk
- www.bma.org.uk
- www.studentmedics.co.uk/medical/
- www.medicalprotection.org/medical_malpractice/medical-student-resources.htm
- www.fleshandbones.com
- www.onexamination.com

The foundation years

9

Dr Rameen Shakur, F2 Academic Medicine Rotation: Cardiology. Nuffield Department of Medicine, the John Radcliffe Hospital, University of Oxford

In this chapter, I would like to share with the reader my own experiences of being a foundation doctor, and what one can expect after graduating from medical school.

The years of hard work at medical school are now behind you. The graduation ceremony seems now to be a distant memory, and all too soon the day that you had once dreamed of when joining medical school is appearing ever closer. Summer is fading and soon August will be upon us.

Those were my thoughts as I pondered about joining as a foundation year 1 doctor, or pre-registration house officer (PRHO) as it was known in the past. The PRHO year was the year prior to gaining full registration with the General Medical Council (GMC). The foundation years continue this tradition, but now, while being provisionally registered with the GMC, one has to undertake a competency-based two-year programme prior to any further specialist postgraduate training. The role of the foundation years is to build and consolidate generic skills that are considered essential to all doctors, regardless of their future speciality. Many of the finer points of this new process continue to evolve and so are beyond the scope of any book. However, much of the process is described in Chapter 11 on career pathways in medicine and surgery.

The move-in

August had begun, and I had moved all my worldly possessions into my room in the designated doctors' flat adjacent to the hospital. Having completed my week of job-shadowing with my predecessor, I was aware of what was being unleashed upon me. I was to take over as the Firm A house officer and at that time become Professor Warrell's and Dr Dwight's houseman at the John Radcliffe. I was excited on the one hand but still anxious nonetheless – for no matter how many weeks I had prepared for this moment, nothing could really prepare me for the first day I entered as a qualified medical graduate. For the first time since embarking on the journey to train as a medic from the sixth form, I was now living the moment – the moment when I wished I could be privileged enough to take care of patients, learn about their disease, be conscientious and compassionate to their holistic needs, and formulate treatment plans in a team setting. Such a sentence seems the sort of thing to use for one's personal statement on the UCAS application form – and probably be asked to explain in an interview. However, those very words came true when I began my first medical job. As my father had told me prior to my joining on my first day, 'Son, welcome to the world of work.'

I had started on my vocation and, as I was to learn during it, work could be both fun and difficult, intriguing and stressful, but never boring.

Having been a student since primary school, one can understand the great transition felt by all medical graduates as for the first time in our lives we are now responsible for not only our own health and safety, but also that of our patients. No more long summer holidays and no more Wednesday afternoons off for sport, we were finally contributing to society after the years of investment by the public.

'Are you the doctor on call?' says the nurse looking after the patient who comes into the medical assessment unit. 'Yes, I am', you answer, and while you wait for that little pat on the back, she quickly answers, 'Hurry up! There are four other patients to see and we have three more expected.' Welcome to a busy teaching hospital!

On-the-job training

As the most junior member of the medical or surgical team, you are expected to do the majority of the administrative as well as the clinical duties relating to a patient's stay in hospital. Often it will be the house officer who will be the first member of the team that a patient will see when arriving at hospital. Thereafter, your seniors will review the patient and optimize or agree with your initial management. Knowledge of the management of acute emergencies is pertinent to a successful foundation year, and slowly but surely you find yourself utilizing those clinical pearls you had learnt while at medical school. In addition, you subconsciously develop your own style of medical practice, which is greatly influenced by how you observe your seniors practise their trade.

Your consultant will play a pivotal role in the early stages of your development. He or she should be responsible for your ongoing clinical training and for providing constant feedback on your performance, even during times when you would rather not hear it!

A team game

It is also vital to have a very good interaction with all other members of your team, such as your registrar, and particularly the nursing and other allied medical staff. A mutually respectful interaction between yourself as the house officer and the nursing staff is essential for a pleasant attachment. There will be times when you will wish bleepers/pagers were never invented. During such stressful times, it is important to remain calm, get through the jobs efficiently and call on your colleagues for help when required. All house officers will have extremely busy periods during their attachment, so it is important that as a group of house officers you all try to help each other out.

The portfolio and continual assessments

One of the major new developments of the foundation programme is the introduction of a portfolio for each house officer. The portfolio is to be used as a record of attainment of competency and to help you plan and manage your foundation programme learning needs. It is envisaged that by identifying areas for development during the programme, you can set out meaningful goals to achieve them. Also, during the programme, you will be assigned a designated educational supervisor (usually your consultant for that attachment), who will be responsible for your educational needs and the attainment of your competencies. All hospitals will have a teaching programme for their house officers. These allocated times should be 'bleep-protected', whereby you are to transfer your bleeper to your senior during the teaching, allowing you to attend the teaching session. Make it a point to attend these sessions, as they are for your benefit.

The tools used to demonstrate your competency to practise as a doctor at your level include the use of formal assessments, as well as gaining feedback from members of your clinical team on your interaction with them and your patients. For formal assessments, senior members of the team (usually, registrars and consultants) should be used during your clinical attachment. To successfully pass each year of your foundation, you must complete a minimum of four to six of each assessment tool to a satisfactory level. The types of formal assessments include:

- **Mini-CEX (Clinical Evaluation Exercise).** This is used to assess your general clinical interaction with your patients. Hence, you will be observed by your assessor during an actual clinical encounter, after which you will be given feedback on your performance. See Figure 1.

- **DOPS (Direct Observation of Procedural Skills).** This is used to assess practical skills such as venepuncture, cannulation and giving intravenous injections. See Figure 2.

- **CbD (Case-based Discussion).** This is used to assess your clinical decision-making skills and the ability to formulate a diagnosis. It is also used by many assessors to further discuss a case that may raise interesting ethical and legal issues. See Figure 3.

Please complete the questions using a cross: ☒   Please use black ink and CAPITAL LETTERS

Doctor's	Surname																											

Forename

GMC Number: **GMC NUMBER MUST BE COMPLETED**

Clinical setting: A&E ☐   OPD ☐   In-patient ☐   Acute Admission ☐   GP Surgery ☐

Clinical problem category: Airway ☐   Breathing ☐   Circulatory ☐   Neuro ☐   Psych/Behav ☐   Pain ☐

New or FU: New ☐   FU ☐   Focus of clinical encounter: History ☐   Diagnosis ☐   Management ☐   Explanation ☐

Number of times patient seen before by trainee: 0 ☐   1-4 ☐   5-9 ☐   >10 ☐

Complexity of case: Low ☐   Average ☐   High ☐   Assessor's position: Consultant ☐   SASG ☐   SpR ☐   GP ☐

Number of previous mini-CEXs observed by assessor with any trainee: 0 ☐   1 ☐   2 ☐   3 ☐   4 ☐   5-9 ☐   >9 ☐

Please grade the following areas using the scale below:	Below expectations for F2 completion		Borderline for F2 completion	Meets expectations for F2 completion	Above expectations for F2 completion		U/C*
	1	2	3	4	5	6	
1 History Taking	☐	☐	☐	☐	☐	☐	☐
2 Physical Examination Skills	☐	☐	☐	☐	☐	☐	☐
3 Communication Skills	☐	☐	☐	☐	☐	☐	☐
4 Clinical Judgement	☐	☐	☐	☐	☐	☐	☐
5 Professionalism	☐	☐	☐	☐	☐	☐	☐
6 Organisation/Efficiency	☐	☐	☐	☐	☐	☐	☐
7 Overall clinical care	☐	☐	☐	☐	☐	☐	☐

*U/C Please mark this if you have not observed the behaviour and therefore feel unable to comment.

Anything especially good?   **Suggestions for development**

Agreed action:

	Not at all									Highly
Trainee satisfaction with mini-CEX	1 ☐	2 ☐	3 ☐	4 ☐	5 ☐	6 ☐	7 ☐	8 ☐	9 ☐	10 ☐
Assessor satisfaction with mini-CEX	1 ☐	2 ☐	3 ☐	4 ☐	5 ☐	6 ☐	7 ☐	8 ☐	9 ☐	10 ☐

Have you had training in the use of this assessment tool?:   ☐ No   ☐ Yes: Written Training   ☐ Yes: Face-to-Face   ☐ Yes: Web/CD rom

Time taken for observation: (in minutes) ☐☐

Assessor's Signature: Date: ☐☐/☐☐/☐☐

Time taken for feedback: (in minutes) ☐☐

Assessor's Surname: 0399259883

Figure 1 Mini-CEX (Clinical Evaluation Exercise) assessment form (reproduced with permission of MMC)

Please complete the questions using a cross: ☒　　Please use black ink and CAPITAL LETTERS

Doctor's Surname

Forename

GMC Number: **GMC NUMBER MUST BE COMPLETED**

Clinical setting: A&E ☐ OPD ☐ In-patient ☐ Acute Admission ☐ GP Surgery ☐

Procedure Number: (Please see guidance) In other please specify:

Assessor's position: Consultant ☐ SASG ☐ SpR ☐ GP ☐ Nurse ☐ Other ☐

Number of previous DOPS observed by assessor with any trainee: 0 ☐ 1 ☐ 2 ☐ 3 ☐ 4 ☐ 5-9 ☐ >9 ☐

Number of times procedure performed by trainee: 0 ☐ 1-4 ☐ 5-9 ☐ >10 ☐ **Difficulty of procedure:** Low ☐ Average ☐ High ☐

Please grade the following areas using the scale below:	Below expectations for F2 completion		Borderline for F2 completion	Meets expectations for F2 completion	Above expectations for F2 completion		U/C*
	1	2	3	4	5	6	
1 Demonstrates understanding of indications, relevant anatomy. technique of procedure	☐	☐	☐	☐	☐	☐	☐
2 Obtains informed consent	☐	☐	☐	☐	☐	☐	☐
3 Demonstrates appropriate preparation pre-procedure	☐	☐	☐	☐	☐	☐	☐
4 Appropriate analgesia or safe sedation	☐	☐	☐	☐	☐	☐	☐
5 Technical ability	☐	☐	☐	☐	☐	☐	☐
6 Aseptic technique	☐	☐	☐	☐	☐	☐	☐
7 Seeks help where appropriate	☐	☐	☐	☐	☐	☐	☐
8 Post procedure management	☐	☐	☐	☐	☐	☐	☐
9 Communication skills	☐	☐	☐	☐	☐	☐	☐
10 Consideration of patient/professionalism	☐	☐	☐	☐	☐	☐	☐
11 Overall ability to perform procedure	☐	☐	☐	☐	☐	☐	☐

*U/C Please mark this if you have not observed the behaviour and therefore feel unable to comment.

Please use this space to record areas of strength or any suggestions for development.

Not at all / Highly
Trainee satisfaction with DOPS 1☐ 2☐ 3☐ 4☐ 5☐ 6☐ 7☐ 8☐ 9☐ 10☐
Assessor satisfaction with DOPS 1☐ 2☐ 3☐ 4☐ 5☐ 6☐ 7☐ 8☐ 9☐ 10☐

Have you had training in the use of this assessment tool?: ☐ No ☐ Yes: Written Training ☐ Yes: Face-to-Face ☐ Yes: Web/CD rom

Time taken for observation: (in minutes)

Assessor's Signature: Date: / /

Time taken for feedback: (in minutes)

Assessor's Surname: 7339084453

Figure 2 DOPS (Direct Observation of Procedural Skills) assessment form (reproduced with permission of MMC)

Please complete the questions using a cross: ☒   Please use black ink and CAPITAL LETTERS

Doctor's	Surname	
	Forename	

GMC Number: **GMC NUMBER MUST BE COMPLETED**

Clinical setting: A&E ☐ OPD ☐ In-patient ☐ Acute Admission ☐ GP Surgery ☐

Clinical problem category: Airway ☐ Breathing ☐ Circulatory ☐ Neuro ☐ Psych/Behav ☐ Pain ☐

Focus of clinical encounter: Medical Record Keeping ☐ Clinical Assessment ☐ Management ☐ Professionalism ☐

Complexity of case: Low ☐ Average ☐ High ☐   Assessor's position: Consultant ☐ SASG ☐ SpR ☐ GP ☐

Please grade the following areas using the scale below:	Below expectations for F2 completion		Borderline for F2 completion	Meets expectations for F2 completion	Above expectations for F2 completion		U/C*
	1	2	3	4	5	6	
1 Medical record keeping	☐	☐	☐	☐	☐	☐	☐
2 Clinical assessment	☐	☐	☐	☐	☐	☐	☐
3 Investigation and referrals	☐	☐	☐	☐	☐	☐	☐
4 Treatment	☐	☐	☐	☐	☐	☐	☐
5 Follow-up and future planning	☐	☐	☐	☐	☐	☐	☐
6 Professionalism	☐	☐	☐	☐	☐	☐	☐
7 Overall clinical judgement	☐	☐	☐	☐	☐	☐	☐

*U/C Please mark this if you have not observed the behaviour and therefore feel unable to comment.

Anything especially good?   **Suggestions for development**

Agreed action:

	Not at all									Highly
Trainee satisfaction with CbD	1 ☐	2 ☐	3 ☐	4 ☐	5 ☐	6 ☐	7 ☐	8 ☐	9 ☐	10 ☐
Assessor satisfaction with CbD	1 ☐	2 ☐	3 ☐	4 ☐	5 ☐	6 ☐	7 ☐	8 ☐	9 ☐	10 ☐

Have you had training in the use of this assessment tool?: ☐ No ☐ Yes: Written Training ☐ Yes: Face-to-Face ☐ Yes: Web/CD rom

Time taken for observation: (in minutes)

Assessor's Signature: Date: Time taken for feedback: (in minutes)

Assessor's Surname:

1058310042

Figure 3 CbD (Case-based Discussion) assessment form (reproduced with permission of MMC)

■ **Mini-PAT (Mini-Peer Assessment Tool)** or **TAB (Team Assessment Behaviour).** This requires you to nominate different members of your clinical team, from supervising consultant to experienced nursing or Allied Health Professional Colleagues, the aim being to better appreciate your interaction within a team setting.

In all cases, the assessment should provide the trainee and the assessor with a means to highlight any areas of improvement and to acknowledge areas of strength. During your attachment, it is best to avoid a last-minute panic in trying to fill these assessments; hence try to complete as many assessments as possible during the attachment itself.

Holidays

Any break, be it a few minutes, hours or days, is a precious commodity for any medical professional. If you are in the privileged position of being able to take your holidays whenever you want, try to space these out throughout your attachment. This will allow you plenty of rest after some busy spells on the wards. Try and enjoy the time off, escaping from medicine for a few days to spend the time with friends and family. It is easy to get 'burnt out' if you try to do too many things while also trying to do clinical duties. Trying to do research, audits and teaching medical students are all great ideas during your foundation year, but it is not necessary to achieve all these goals in just the one attachment. There is time throughout the foundation programme to do these and to take advantage of other educational opportunities you may be interested in. The appropriate time for each should be discussed with your educational supervisor, who can advise you on how to space out your time effectively.

Enjoy the time

I learnt a lot and enjoyed my time as a F1 doctor. The learning curve is very steep initially, as you are faced with this new-found responsibility. However, compared with the past, support for junior members of the team has greatly improved. You are also no longer expected to work ridiculous hours and to be sleep-deprived for months on end. Yet, this does not mean that your time will not be busy or stressful – it will be, but it is important to keep things in perspective and seek help early if you should feel things are getting too much for you. You are a vital member of the team. As my previous consultant said, 'The house officer is the lynchpin of the medical team.' Having passed your final medical school exams, you have already proved that you are a capable member of the medical profession. The foundation years are there to provide you with the skills needed to progress in postgraduate medicine. Therefore enjoy the time and make the most of your opportunities.

Summary

▓ The role of the foundation years is to build and consolidate generic skills that are considered essential for all medical doctors, regardless of their future speciality.

▓ It is also vital to have good interaction with all other members of your team, in particular, your registrar and the nursing and allied medical staff.

▓ The portfolio is to be used as a record of attainment of competency and to help you plan and manage your foundation programme learning needs.

▓ For formal assessments, senior members of the team (registrars and consultants) should be used during your clinical attachment.

▓ Any break, be it a few minutes, hours or days, is a precious commodity for any house officer.

▓ The learning curve is very steep initially, as you are faced with this new-found responsibility.

▓ Enjoy the time and make the most of your opportunities.

Choosing general practice (primary care) 10

Dr Edward Shaoul, Honorary Senior Lecturer, Imperial College London

This chapter will discuss the entry requirements for general practice (primary care), and will focus on what this branch of medicine can offer you and what opportunities are made available from it.

Medical school entry

If you already feel a strong vocation towards general practice (primary care) and wish to say so at your selection interview, there is no harm in doing so. These days, general practitioners (GPs) sit on many interview panels, and it will be recognized by the interviewers that the initial aspirations of most candidates will change in the course of their career.

The medical school curriculum is as comprehensive as possible. There will be many opportunities to see most specialties, including general practice (primary care), in the course of the five or six years that you will be at medical school, and many undergraduates become tempted by what they see changing in a positive and healthy way throughout their undergraduate years. However, about 60% of all undergraduates in medicine will make a career in general practice (primary care) for a variety of reasons.

Reasons for choosing general practice (primary care)

There is an opportunity to see a wide range of conditions in which you will be the first-in-line doctor, which can be very exciting. More than 90% of patients who consult a GP will be managed and treated within the primary care setting. You will have the opportunity to provide continuity of care and be able to see the progress or cure of a particular condition. You will form a relationship within the community in which you work, and will enjoy independence as a self-employed practitioner who, in fact, will employ staff to work with him.

A few practitioners choose to be employed within a small-organization setting; it seems likely that about 30% of GPs will choose this route in the future. However, as a self-employed doctor, you will be able to exercise more control over the hours of work, allowing considerable freedom with the organization of family life – this is particularly helpful to those doctors in the childbearing years.

The entrance conditions are shorter and less arduous than for many other specialties. As a result, you will reach a responsible status earlier and will have the opportunity to work longer, so that your lifelong earnings will be comparable to those of doctors who choose to go into a hospital specialty.

There will be ample opportunity for you to become an expert in a particular field if you wish to do so, and to temper the work that you do with patients with other activities – this may be professional or non-professional.

General practice (primary care) entry

The basic medical degree and hospital officer posts are common to all branches of medicine. Undergraduates who have attained and developed a broad view are likely to be successful in entering general practice (primary care) training schemes. Do not be frightened to continue to practise your music, develop your dramatic skills, work abroad in medicine for a short period of time or spend a year doing a research post.

Once you have completed your foundation training, you can apply at any time for a speciality training scheme in general practice (primary care), previously called the vocational training scheme. This will guarantee a complete training package without needing to find a new hospital post every six months or a general practice (primary care) registrarship. Most of these posts are at post foundation level and are usually based at one deanery. There will be a special training programme for general practice (primary care) in addition to the specialty teaching programme.

Entry requirements for the scheme will encompass recent changes to national speciality and GP training by MMC. More information is provided in Chapter 11 on career pathways in medicine and surgery.

General practice (primary care) training is well organized and well monitored. The hospital posts and general practice (primary care) training posts are selected with great care and are constantly supervised. The programme is run at a local level by a course organizer, who will work at a personal level with all doctors on the scheme.

To complete the training period, doctors must pass a coursework examination called Summative Assessment, which tests their clinical knowledge and skills together with their consultation skills. This is set at a minimal competence level so that any doctor who has been admitted to the training course, and applies him or herself diligently, should be able to pass.

An alternative assessment by examination for Membership of the Royal College of General Practitioners is also available. This is likely to become the normal route of entry in the future.

Work involved in general practice (primary care)

What do GPs do? Why is it exciting? Is it financially rewarding? What other benefits are there? These questions are answered in this section.

The patients you see as a GP are not selected by another professional. You find that your day is made up of a mix of very common and extremely rare conditions. This requires you to possess very highly refined diagnostic skills and to be able to recognize small differences between apparently similar presentations. You will have ample opportunity to use a variety of personal skills in areas such as psychiatry, manipulation, skin conditions, surgical conditions and eye examinations, and you will be able to recognize your particular skills and interests and have the opportunity to expand such skills.

You will be in a unique position to view the whole patient and understand any underlying problems, not just necessarily make a clinical diagnosis. You will work not only with individual patients, but also with their families who may be registered with you. You will be able to see patients as frequently as you think necessary, you will be able to visit them at their home, and they will feel able and comfortable to approach you in a non-formal manner. You will thus be able to develop knowledge of the whole family structure, which may include anything up to five generations of one family. You will witness family life events such as births, marriages and, sadly, deaths.

In addition to your day-to-day contact with your patients, you will have ample opportunity from general practice (primary care) to develop related interests. These may be academic interests, helping to teach undergraduates and postgraduates the various skills of general practice (primary care); being involved in research, either on your own or as part of a team; developing an interest in forensic medicine, such as police work; or choosing to make an in-depth study of family dynamics and family medicine. Some of you will use general practice (primary care) as a base to develop your interests in occupational health. A few of you will develop such skills and interests and will continue to do either one or two hospital sessions per week in certain specialties, such as dermatology, psychiatry, and accident and emergency. An increasing number of GPs provide a service within their primary care organization for other practices in areas such as anticoagulation, minor surgery, dermatology and heart failure diagnosis. Most of these additional interests carry a financial reward.

General practice (primary care) versus hospital medicine

You have to admit that general practice (primary care) sounds very exciting and stimulating, but, for example, how does the pay compare with that of specialist colleagues? It is important to remember that GPs start earning a full income sooner than their hospital colleagues do, and can also work for as long as they wish. There is no compulsory retirement age, although GPs have to show that they are competent. Demonstration of competence will be normal throughout all medical careers. The method of assessment has still not been determined.

General practice (primary care) income has become very variable. Some doctors will be content to work in a controlled environment earning about £80 000 (2006 figures). Others will be happy to take on the responsibilities of partnership and earn up to twice that figure. This recent change has meant that GPs' income is considerably in excess of their consultant colleagues.

Some hospital specialists will develop a lucrative private practice, and there is no denying that those who work very hard will achieve extremely high levels of earning. Many hospital specialists will be able, at some time in their career, to receive a boost to their income called the merit award, but there is no equivalent scheme for general practice (primary care). However, GPs have the opportunity to invest in their surgery premises at favourable rates, and many find that they are able to make a capital gain when they come to retire from general practice (primary care).

Hospital doctors are employed by the Health Service Trust for which they work. The Trust will provide them with a fixed income and will be responsible for the equipment they use and the staff they have to support them. The Trust will also expect the doctors they employ to be managed by managers employed by the Trust. The structure in general practice (primary care) is very different. The contract offered by the health authority to GPs is fixed centrally and can be changed arbitrarily by the government. Nevertheless, GPs remain independent contractors and can choose their level of work and the patients for whom they wish to be responsible. Freedom of choice in the management of certain conditions is possible. Although some doctors will choose to provide care for drug addicts on their list, others may decide that this is not an aspect of general practice (primary care) that they enjoy and may exclude such care from their contract.

There is also an opportunity to vary the length of the working week in general practice (primary care), and, because of their independence, GPs can rearrange their workload within the practice, organize their holidays, choose their professional partners and, very importantly, choose the staff they wish to employ. Since the introduction of the new contract in 2004, very few urban doctors work out of hours and weekends. The work is undertaken by the Primary Care Organization currently, for a fee of 6% of the GP's income. Many practitioners own the premises in which they work, and, in recognizing the importance of satisfactory working conditions for general practice (primary care), the Department of Health have a number of supportive financial schemes to enable practices to build new premises and renovate old premises.

It is important to understand that all branches of medicine are challenging, and if you are in doubt as to whether or not you can meet these demands, it is probably better not to start. In addition, you should be aware that you can succeed in any branch of medicine you choose if you want to. You will change your mind several times on the way through medical school and in the early years of your career – some doctors even change their minds much later on. Between 50% and 60% of all entrants will become GPs.

Types of practice

Single-handed practice

Some doctors who enter general practice (primary care) do not enjoy working in partnership with other doctors for a variety of reasons. This is very often due to a financial dispute that has arisen in a previous partnership arrangement. It may also be because the doctor concerned has found it difficult to find colleagues with whom they can work, and prefers the ease of decision-making involved in working single-handed. There are no long practice meetings for them and no need to bend their wishes to those of other partners. However, a disadvantage to working in a single-handed practice is that you are isolated, both professionally and in the provision of cover for absence. There are many ways to overcome this disadvantage, and many single-handed practitioners work in close cooperation with other single-handed practitioners to obtain some of the benefits of working together without the administrative difficulties that arise from partnerships.

Partnership

Most GPs will work in partnership, and the trend over the past 10 years has been for these partnerships to become bigger and bigger. By pooling resources, these practices are able to buy equipment needed to help in their daily work and to employ a practice manager to help to take some of the administrative burden off their shoulders. They are also often able to have a wider variety of practice staff working with them and to be able to host educational meetings within their premises.

Increasingly, partnerships are employing doctors who wish to restrict their responsibilities or hours, providing a guaranteed income and a safe environment in which to work. There need be no long-term commitment to stay in the same practice. This arrangement seems to suit the needs of some doctors.

Health centres

A few practices will choose to work from Health Service-owned premises called health centres. They are spared the financial responsibility for the building from which they work, and have the benefit of working in close proximity with other healthcare workers employed by the community trust but not by the practice. Many practitioners have learnt that the quality of these buildings often leaves a lot to be desired, and the maintenance often requires protracted negotiation with the financially restricted Health Authority that is responsible for maintaining them. So most practitioners prefer to work from modern, privately developed premises for which they receive considerable financial support from the Health Service, but with the partners retaining the independence that comes from owning the building, together with the opportunities to make a capital gain in later life.

Location of practice

Where do doctors choose to practise? In the case of partners, there are three distinct areas. Some doctors will choose to work a long way away from cities and to set up practice in a rural area. Although these are often geographically very desirable and provide an excellent quality of life, they can be very demanding, requiring a high level of interventional skills to compensate for the distance to the nearest hospital, and there are difficulties of professional isolation because of the distance between the various doctors who are working together.

In contrast, some doctors may choose to work in an inner-city practice where the entire practice population is within half a mile. In these practices, you would need to meet the challenges of a multicultural society, bringing with it language difficulties for some patients, and often very specialized populations, such as a refugee population. This is compensated for by being near hospitals, often teaching hospitals with ample opportunities to learn new skills and to be heavily involved in the teaching of undergraduate students from those hospitals.

Somewhere between these two extremes are the practices working in the leafy suburbs, often with very comfortable premises, not too far from the main hospitals and with an excellent community relationship with the local hospital – many doctors opt to work in such an area. However, nothing is completely idyllic, and patients living in these areas are often very demanding and cause the doctors a considerable amount of frustration.

Increasingly, we are now finding that many younger doctors are choosing not to commit themselves to a lifelong attachment to a particular practice. They are not opting to go into partnership, but rather to work within practices as assistants or as salaried principals. These doctors will earn less money and will not be entitled to the tax advantages of being self-employed, but they will often find the comfort of having a guaranteed income adequate compensation for this. What I have tried to show you is that the opportunities that exist are very varied.

Typical working day in general practice (primary care)

What is a day in general practice (primary care) like? What is the nature of the work? Why do I find it attractive and so rewarding? I will outline my typical day to help answer these questions and to give an insight into general practice (primary care).

The day starts with morning surgery. In addition to the patients who have made appointments, there will usually be an extra three or four who feel their condition so urgent that they cannot wait for the next surgery. Some of these patients will have a minor problem that can easily be dismissed by reassurance or confirmation of a simple diagnosis such as mumps or chickenpox. Occasionally, among these extra patients, there will be one that constitutes a real emergency, which could be a severe asthma attack, a heart attack or bleeding from somewhere in the gastrointestinal tract. You will be faced with the difficulty of dealing with this emergency, knowing that those patients who have booked a routine appointment will inevitably be seen later than they had expected. Nevertheless, the satisfactory management of the emergency not only helps the patient concerned but also gives the doctor considerable satisfaction. Perhaps not surprisingly, the patients who were delayed in the waiting room are usually very understanding and grateful that it was not their emergency with which you were having to deal.

The variety in the morning surgery will be infinite. A few of the patients will be undergoing routine monitoring procedures for reasonably well-controlled hypertension or diabetes, but every so often one patient will be completely out of control and all your skill will be needed. You may well be within a small influenza epidemic and seeing half a dozen patients with coughs, colds and bad chests, and yet you will have the responsibility of picking out among those patients the one who has tuber- 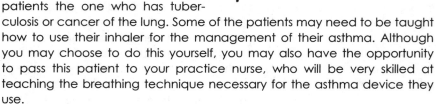 culosis or cancer of the lung. Some of the patients may need to be taught how to use their inhaler for the management of their asthma. Although you may choose to do this yourself, you may also have the opportunity to pass this patient to your practice nurse, who will be very skilled at teaching the breathing technique necessary for the asthma device they use.

A patient may present with recurring headaches. You will be aware from the knowledge of the family of a number of background problems to be overcome in order to resolve the symptoms. You will then call in the next patient. Their face will be all smiles as they come to thank you for correctly diagnosing the lump in their breast as having been a very early cancer that had been successfully removed at the local breast clinic, giving the patient a clean bill of health.

At the end of the morning surgery, I may well go on to run my antenatal clinic, regrettably no longer in conjunction with one of the midwives from the local hospital. Some of the mothers that I will be examining will be the very babies that I delivered at home or in a hospital unit 25 years ago. Other mothers will be new to me, and I will need to establish with them the strong family links that I consider to be important to my style of practice. An antenatal clinic is very different from morning surgery. The patients are well, they are happy, they are a little bit anxious but easily reassured, and it is great fun demonstrating to them the various bits of the baby's anatomy that can be felt through the abdominal wall. They have many questions to ask, but somehow this never seems to be a chore. The morning is all too short, and it is already time to stop for lunch.

Sometimes lunch will mean jumping in the car and driving to a meeting and eating sandwiches while matters of Health Service administration are discussed at one committee or another, or perhaps the teaching of medical students for the forthcoming term. Sometimes, lunch is meeting with the partners and perhaps part of the practice team to discuss the running of the practice itself. Sometimes, it is a personal affair with nothing to disturb the flow of digestive juices.

I find nowadays that I can very rarely do any home visits in the morning, so I will plan to do these in the afternoon. Most visits these days will involve seeing patients who have no mobility at all. The majority of patients now come to the practice. However, one group of patients that I do choose to visit at home are mothers who have just had a baby. I find that it helps considerably in the development of a close relationship between the practice and the mothers, and it gives me an opportunity to meet them in their home surroundings, where they can proudly show me their baby. I can answer their many questions about the management of this new member of their family. I will then go back to the surgery and read the not inconsiderable quantity of mail that has arrived and make decisions on the results of pathological tests that have been returned to me. I may have discussions with the district nurses or the practice nurses about procedures that need to be carried out, and will then start the evening surgery, which in many ways will be similar to the morning surgery, although the mix of patients and the pace of the surgery are often very different. At the end of the day, I will ensure that all the actions that I needed to take for that day have been completed and go home.

It used to be that going home meant going home to be on duty for the practice. However, with the advent of the new contract (2004), we can now go home knowing that we will not be disturbed. Although this change in working pattern is relatively recent, it became inevitable with the increasing workload in the daytime. Also, the increasing demands of patients for out-of-hours attention coupled with an increasing expectation of young practitioners for a more satisfactory quality of family life, which they found they were having difficulty in protecting, led to this change.

Is it worthwhile?

It is probably true to say that every day that I work in my surgery there will be at least one event that leads me to say, 'I am glad that I went to work today and was able to do something to help a particular patient.' You certainly do not get up in the morning looking for that gratification, but, nevertheless, when it happens, it increases the fun of general practice (primary care).

Summary

■ More than 90% of patients who consult a GP will be managed and treated within the primary-care setting.

■ Once you have completed your registration, you can at any time apply for a three-year rotation for general practice (primary care), called the vocational training scheme.

■ You will be in a unique position to view the whole patient and understand any underlying problems, not just necessarily make a clinical diagnosis.

■ Most GPs will work in partnership, and the trend over the past 10 years has been for these partnerships to become bigger and bigger.

Further reading

Brewster B, Mills J. *The Doctor*. London: BBC, 1991.

Humphries J, Brown L. *Careers in Medicine, Dentistry and Mental Health*. London: Kogan Page, 1996.

Richards P, Stockill S, Foster R *et al*. *Learning Medicine*. Cambridge: Cambridge University Press, 2006.

RCGP Careers Information Pack. This can be obtained from 14 Princes Gate, Hyde Park, London SW7 1PU or www.rcgp.org.uk.

www.bma.org.uk/ap.nsf/Content/NewGMScontract/$file/gpcont.pdf.

Career pathways in medicine and surgery

11

Dr Yasir Al-Wakeel, F2 Academic Medicine Rotation, Nuffield Department of Medicine, the John Radcliffe Hospital, University of Oxford
Mr Ashok Handa, Honorary Consultant Vascular Surgeon and Clinical Tutor in Surgery, Nuffield Department of Surgery, the John Radcliffe Hospital, University of Oxford

You have sat your medical finals and the powers that be (the General Medical Council) have decided that you are fit to practise as a doctor and have awarded you provisional registration. So what comes next?

This chapter explores the options available to medical graduates upon starting work within the NHS and the current government plans for career progression in the medical profession. As medical career pathways are currently undergoing constant evolution, readers are requested to stay abreast of the latest changes in the system through visiting the MMC website on: www.mmc.nhs.uk/.

Postgraduate training in the UK is currently undergoing substantial change. The NHS, under the MMC (Modernising Medical Careers) flagship, aims to improve patient care by delivering a modernized and focused career structure for doctors. Thus, from August 2005, all newly qualified doctors embarked on a two-year foundation programme.[1]

The Postgraduate Medical Education and Training Board

Postgraduate training is overseen by the Postgraduate Medical Education and Training Board (PMETB), which from September 2005 took over from the Specialty Training Authority and the Joint Committee on Postgraduate Training for General Practice. As one overall body responsible for both specialist training and general practice, its main remit is that of medical training, and it is charged with the role of approving training programmes. PMETB, the Royal Colleges and the Regional Postgraduate Dean are responsible for ensuring standards and determining curricula.

The foundation programme

This is a two-year programme that aims to bridge the gap between medical school and specialist/general practice training. The main difference between the first foundation year (F1) and the old Pre-Registration

House Officer (PRHO) year will be the emphasis upon demonstrating competence in a variety of skills thought to be essential for attaining full registration with the GMC. While most of the old PRHO jobs consisted of two six-month rotations, a typical F1 year may involve three sets of four-month placements in specialties such as general medicine, general surgery and paediatrics. Having completed the tasks set out in the F1 curriculum, while keeping an up-to-date portfolio, full GMC registration will be awarded after completion of the F1 year.

Throughout both F1 and F2, you will rotate, mostly, through four-month rotations that will provide you with key competencies in dealing with the acutely ill patient as well as developing effective team-working and communication skills. At least one of the placements is likely to be in a community setting, for example general practice, community paediatrics or community psychiatry. This may be particularly useful for those intending to work in hospital medicine, for whom this may be the only chance they have to experience work in the community setting. Rotations are also likely to be spread out between large teaching hospitals and smaller district general hospitals. Both environments have their advantages, and disadvantages, and so decisions regarding location are often dictated by personal reasons.

The two-year foundation programme will also allow you to gain insight into your future career path. For some, a stint in public health may open their eyes to a specialty they would not otherwise have considered. Alternatively, you may have already decided that you want to be a surgeon, in which case more surgically inclined specialties in F2 will be a bonus. However, as the foundation scheme seeks to develop generic broad-based skills, there is consensus that appointment to specialist training should not be contingent on time spent in that specialty during the foundation programme. There is also consensus that gaining college examinations (e.g. MRCP or MRCS) during F2 would detract from the learning objectives of the foundation programme.

The run-through grade

Higher specialist training used to take place via the Specialist Registrar (SpR) post. This system, known as the Calman system, often resulted in a considerable wait between gaining membership exams as a Senior House Officer (SHO) and gaining a National Training Number (NTN) allowing one to become a SpR.

The run-through grade effectively combines basic (SHO) and higher specialist (SpR) training in an effort to circumvent the unforeseen effects of the Calman system. The run-through grade promises seamless progression from foundation programme to specialist training, a reduction of bottlenecks and non-standard posts, and greater career flexibility.[2]

There will be two main types of run-through grade:

▓ specialty entry
▓ broad-based entry.

A variety of specialties intend to select trainees straight from foundation level to specific run-through programmes. These include general practice, histopathology, urology and the neurosciences. On the other hand, many Royal Colleges will be implementing a broad-based entry approach leading to a wide range of specialist training outcomes. This would mean that if, for example, you wanted to do medicine, you would start a medicine run-through grade that initially focused on a broad range of medical specialties, following which you could either specialize in general medicine or complete the run-through grade in a chosen specialty. This approach would be in line with the fact that up to 60% of UK medical graduates are undecided about their final career path 18 months after qualifying.[3] Furthermore, there will be competitive opportunities for trainees in specialist training to move between programmes according to service or personal need. Figure 1 illustrates the current shape of career pathways.

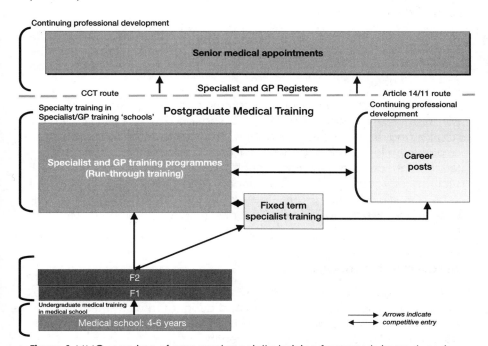

Figure 1 MMC overview of proposed specialty training framework (reproduced with permission of MMC)

Medicine

The Federation of the Royal Colleges of Physicians has proposed a system whereby those wanting to train in a medical specialty, as well as others who consider basic medical training a good foundation for other career paths, apply for Basic Medical Training (BMT) years 1 and 2. These years would encompass four-month blocks of specialties, including geriatrics, accident and emergency, intensive treatment unit, and others, to form a broad base of acute medicine on which to build more specialized training. Following this, applicants would compete for entry into Higher Specialist Training (HST) years 1–4 in their chosen specialty. The Royal College of Physicians is also keen to establish acute medicine as a specialty in its own right via BMT 1 and 2 followed by three years of higher specialist training.

Competitive entry to BMT is likely to take place via a national scheme that would match trainee choices for a preferred specialty and geographical area. It is likely that ranking in the exam for membership of the Royal College of Physicians (MRCP), combined with portfolios and objective structured clinical exam (OSCE)-type interviews, will form the basis for selection.

Surgery

MMC has also meant an overhaul of surgical selection and career structure. With the number of applicants for each post set to increase with the influx of European and other overseas graduates, selection needs to be open and objective.

After the two-year foundation programme, the third postgraduate year will form the first year of surgical training and will consist of general surgery and other surgical specialties. This stand-alone year will be an opportunity to develop generic surgical competencies and prepare for the forthcoming selection. Specific courses should be completed, such as advanced trauma life support (ATLS), and, halfway into the year, a multiple-choice exam – likely to be the Part 1 exam for membership of the Royal College of Surgeons (MRCS) – will be taken and ranked.

Assessment centres

At the end of the year, candidates will apply via a University and Colleges Admissions Service (UCAS)-type form and designated assessment centres. Application forms are likely to include ranked MRCS result, the candidate's portfolio, and their ranked selection of four specialties and four localities. The top third or so will be invited to the assessment centres to undertake a barrage of cognitive tests and tests of hand–eye coordination and decision-making under stress, replacing the reliance on academic record.

Interviews

In addition to these objective assessments of professional skills, candidates will take part in structured interviews. It is envisaged that those not selected for assessment will use the skills acquired to bolster their portfolios for application to other specialties, such as gynaecology and interventional radiology. Surgical training years 2–6 or 7 would then form higher surgical training.

Accreditation

Upon satisfactory completion of the run-through grade, candidates will be accredited with the Certificate of Completion of Training (CCT), a common certificate of training for all doctors (specialists and general practitioners). In some specialties, according to service need and following open competition, it may be possible to extend the CCT to incorporate specific subspecialist training, although this is likely to be in far smaller numbers than those obtaining a CCT.

Academic medicine

All doctors need a firm grounding in science, and will need to develop the requisite skills of critically appraising scientific papers. The move towards evidence-based medicine, that is to say, making treatment decisions based upon data from clinical trials, makes keeping abreast of research essential. However, some doctors will choose to take a more active role in research, often combining clinical commitments with those of running clinical trials.

And yet, despite an increase in medical student numbers, the number of clinical academics has declined steadily over the past five years. Part of the problem stemmed from the lack of a clear route of entry and a transparent career structure. Furthermore, clinical academics have traditionally had to fulfil multiple roles, including researcher, teacher, clinician and administrator. These 'jacks of all trades' also lacked pay parity with their full-time NHS counterparts.

These issues are being tackled head on by MMC. Academic foundation posts, which can take the form of either an integrated approach encompassing academic activities throughout the year or a four-month block within the foundation years, are designed to be a stepping stone for a defined specialist route (Figure 2).[4] Host institutions will compete for about

INTEGRATED ACADEMIC TRAINING PATH

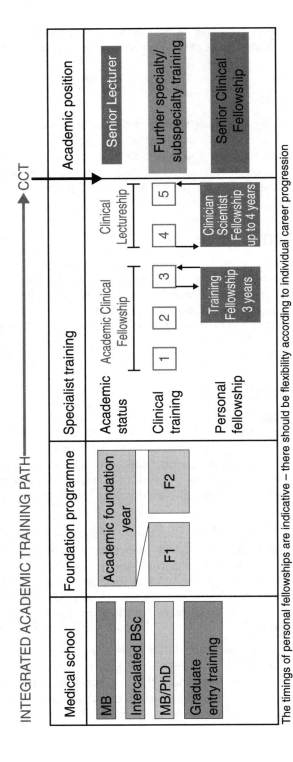

The timings of personal fellowships are indicative – there should be flexibility according to individual career progression

Figure 2 Proposed framework for academic training. From Report of the Academic Sub-committee of MMC and the UK CRC (reproduced with permission of MMC)

100 dedicated academic run-through grade posts, which will be centrally funded. The academic run-through grade is divided into two parts: the Academic Clinical Fellowship phase leading to a Training Fellowship and a higher degree, and the Clinical Lectureship phase leading to the CCT. This is likely to take two years longer than the corresponding clinical run-through grade.

Summary

- Only time will tell whether or not MMC will succeed. The promise of streamlined training and a consultant-led NHS can only be good for both the medical profession and the public.

- The proposed reduction in years spent training (already being limited by the European Working Time Directive), may mean that at the end of the run-through grade you are a Junior Consultant – equivalent to the old Senior Registrar.

- Despite the promise of broad-based entry and the ability to transfer from one specialist training scheme to another, it is likely that those who are decided on their choice of career will benefit when it comes to specialist selection under MMC.

- Tomorrow's doctor will be both dynamic and adaptable to the needs of an ever-changing workforce.

- However, with over 60 specialties to choose from, medicine does not lack variety.

References

1. Al-Wakeel Y, Handa A. Foundation and beyond: Is the future any clearer? *BMJ Career Focus* 2006; **332**: 3–5.

2. British Medical Association Junior Doctors Committee. *The Shape of Specialist Training – Aspirations for Seamless Progression*. London: BMA, 2005 (www.bma.org.uk/ap.nsf/Content/shapeofspclsttraining/$file/TheShape.pdf).

3. BMA Graduate Cohort Study, 2005 (www.bma.org.uk/ap.nsf/Content/shapeofspclsttraining/$file/TheShape.pdf).

4. Report of the Academic Sub-committee of Modernising Medical Careers and the UK Clinical Research Collaboration. *Medically and Dentally Qualified Academic Staff: Recommendations for Training the Researchers and Educators of the Future*, 2005 (www.mmc.nhs.uk/download_files/Overview-of-proposed-specialty-training-framework1.doc).

Choosing hospital medicine 12

Dr Paul Ayuk, Former Clinical Lecturer in Obstetrics and Gynaecology, the John Radcliffe Hospital, University of Oxford

When you graduate from medical school, you will be given the title of medical doctor. This title carries a status within society, and there is an expectation from the public about what you should be able to do – make a diagnosis and treat the sick. This is traditionally known as 'doctoring'.

You will quickly recognize that there is a lot more that a medical graduate can do in addition to or apart from 'doctoring' while contributing to the care of patients within the hospital. This chapter aims to explore the options open to one as a hospital doctor.

Career pathways

The career pathways within hospital medicine have changed substantially over the last 10 years, and continue to change. The details may therefore be slightly different by the time you graduate. Following graduation, you will be required to undergo two years of foundation training (F1 and F2). These are highly structured programmes with specific training objectives and regular appraisals. Following this, those choosing a career in hospital medicine will have to enter a specialist training programme. Currently, this is represented by the Specialist Registrar training programme but most specialties are likely to require additional training before the equivalent of the Specialist Registrar grade is attained. Entry into specialist training will be by open competition, usually in the form of a job application form and interview. At the end of specialist training (about 5 years), you will be qualified to enter the Specialist Register and apply for a consultant post.

For more information, see Chapter 11 on career pathways in medicine and surgery.

Teamwork in hospital medicine

The working pattern of hospital doctors has changed considerably, and many doctors in training now do shift work. This means that you may do a night shift (say, midnight to 8 AM) for one week and then do a different shift the following week, with an appropriate rest period. For effective patient care, it is vital that all medical professionals recognize and fulfil their roles within the team that is on duty. Many specialties have retained a consultant-led team structure, where every doctor belongs to a team led by a consultant or group of consultants with ultimate responsibility for a group of patients. To be effective, you have to be able to communicate with other members of the team.

There are, however, a large number of other professionals who contribute to and take responsibility for the care of patients. These include nurses, midwives, physiotherapists, social workers, speech therapists and many more. One of the most important skills you will need to acquire during your medical school training is knowing when to call for assistance and the most appropriate person to call. You therefore need to be able to work closely and communicate with other medical professionals.

Many patients in hospital have more than one disease or may develop other conditions while in hospital. It is therefore very common for the junior doctor to be required to refer a patient to or ask for advice from another specialist or from a colleague within the same specialty. Finally, you may need to obtain more information from or send information to the patient's general practitioner. Again, you will need to be able to communicate effectively and 'sell your case' while being absolutely accurate. It is amazing how some junior doctors can always manage to get their patients seen immediately, while others have to wait several days for a review by another specialist.

Finally, the most important member of the team is actually the patient (and their family). The days when doctors decided what was best for the patient and treated them in their best interest are thankfully long gone. All patients should now be involved in making decisions about their care and should be given sufficient information to help them make decisions. Communication with patients and their families is increasingly important in medicine, and good communication skills are essential to be an effective doctor.

Quality of life and hospital medicine

The last 10 years have seen substantial changes in the quality of life of junior hospital doctors, and possibly of consultants as well. The days when junior hospital doctors were contracted to work 72 hours a week and regularly worked for longer have long gone. A career in hospital medicine is, however, challenging, and you will usually need to spend a lot of your spare time studying in order to succeed.

Competition

Like any other profession, hospital medicine is very competitive, and the level of competition varies between different specialties and with time within a particular specialty. One is most likely to face particularly stiff competition at three levels.

Passing postgraduate exams

Every specialty has exams (usually two, but sometimes three) that you must pass in order to become a specialist in that field. These exams are administered by a Royal College; for instance, the Royal College of Obstetricians and Gynaecologists and the Royal College of Physicians will administer exams for obstetricians and gynaecologists and for physicians respectively. Most colleges apply 'standard setting' to their exams, and this means that you may score, say, 79% in an exam and still not pass.

Obtaining a Specialist Registrar training post

The government estimates how many consultants it requires in any particular specialty and then creates an appropriate number of training posts, which are divided amongst the different deaneries (or regions of the country). There are always more applicants than there are training posts, and competition for these is usually very stiff. This means that you may be a perfectly good doctor and qualified to have a training post, but there may not be enough to go round or there are others who are better qualified than you and/or have waited for longer.

Obtaining a consultant position

Becoming a consultant is the ultimate intention of all those embarking on a career in hospital medicine. Once appointed, most consultants are in post until they retire (usually about 25–30 years), and unless a new post is created, a particular job will only be available every 25 years or so. While competition is usually stiff, you have to be certain that you will want to spend the rest of your working life in that particular hospital and possibly bring up your family in that part of the country. It is therefore easy to see why some jobs in some parts of the country will be highly sought after. (For an example of the daily duties of a consultant see the appendix to this chapter).

However, given the changes in medical careers, only time will tell as to where the new challenges lie for doctors of differing specialties. (See also Chapter 11 on career pathways in medicine and surgery.)

Flexibility

You may be left with the impression that once you are signed up to a training programme, you will be told where to work, when and for how long. To a certain extent, this is accurate, as there has to be a degree of management and control for any such system to be effective. However, there is some flexibility, and you will need to learn how to use the system to your advantage. There is also some flexibility regarding what you do outside the training programme, but again there are limits to ensure that you qualify with an appropriate level of competence. Some individuals spend part of their training in centres of excellence abroad, and this may bring new skills and expertise into the country. In my department, recently, I shared an office with a colleague who had spent two years working as a medical director for an Internet company before returning to complete his specialist training. The skills he brought into the department meant that within two years of his appointment, he had dramatically improved the way we taught, examined and communicated with medical students by introducing web-based learning, building the websites himself. Another colleague had spent two years as a management consultant in the City. During my training, I developed a website which has trained over 1000 doctors taking their postgraduate exams in obstetrics and gynaecology in three years from over 15 countries. Having completed my specialist training, I have taken time off to spend time with my 17-month-old son! Such career choices are increasingly common in hospital medicine, and demonstrate that you can have a life and still be a dedicated and successful hospital doctor.

Research

You will quickly realize that there are many diseases whose causes we do not know or for which we do not have effective treatment. In addition, there are always new diseases for which the cause and treatments have to be found. Most of this work is done by scientists – people with training in basic science subjects such as biochemistry, physiology and molecular biology. However, these scientists do not usually have access to patients, while the doctors who have access to patients do not usually have the scientific knowledge to do the experiments to find new treatments. The easy answer is for medical doctors and scientists to work together – and such teamwork or collaboration is usually very effective. However, it will be more efficient if the medical knowledge, access to patients and scientific expertise were available in the same individual. Being a medical doctor and doing basic scientific research at the same time is a fascinating experience, and will suit those who have a thirst for knowledge and the enthusiasm to go and look for answers. Almost everyone who is a professor in a hospital would have had some basic scientific training.

There are some disadvantages to being a researcher. The training is longer and harder, as you will need to train in treating patients to the same level as everyone else and train in basic science research to a similar level as scientists. You will also have to divide your time between seeing patients and doing research, and this means that you probably will not be as good at these things as those who see patients, do operations or do scientific research all the time. You will usually depend on money from charities to do your research, and this can be frustrating. Finally, the discoveries that you make may take a long time before being translated into drugs or treatments that improve patient care. However, basic scientific research is the only way by which we can keep discovering new treatments, and the rewards to the individual and the patients far outweigh any drawbacks. (See also Chapter 15 on academic medicine.)

Teaching

All hospital doctors are involved in teaching – usually their colleagues or medical students, but sometimes also nurses, midwives and other medical professionals. Unlike most of the teachers in your school, who have a teaching qualification in addition to their university degree, most doctors who teach have very little formal training and do not have any recognized teaching qualifications. However, doctors with an interest in teaching can acquire the necessary qualifications, and these individuals usually make a difference to teaching methods in their departments and therefore to the quality of the medical students and junior doctors who pass through those departments. In this way, a single individual can influence the quality of a large number of doctors and therefore the outcome of a large number of patients. It is vital that medicine attract young people with an interest in teaching and the enthusiasm to acquire the necessary training.

Summary

- In the past, hospital medicine was regarded as a hard slog – and to an extent it still is, given that you will be dealing with the lives of individuals and families.

- With recent changes in training and working hours, a career in hospital medicine brings enormous personal satisfaction from seeing the improvements in the lives and health of individuals and families.

- The lifestyle and income are not bad either!

Appendix: A week in the life of a consultant physician

Dr Hywel Jones, Consultant Physician and District Clinical Tutor, the John Radcliffe Hospital, Oxford

There is no such thing as a typical working week for a consultant physician. There will be fixed commitments such as outpatients and ward rounds occurring at the same time each week, but the patients will always have a variety of different problems and diseases that have to be addressed. It is this variety and complexity of problems that make a career in medicine both rewarding and challenging. In addition to looking after patients in the outpatient clinic and on the wards, there is the opportunity to deal with emergency medical admissions, including patients with heart attacks, strokes and infections, as well as patients who present with illnesses where the diagnosis is not obvious but has to be made by the physicians, often in close collaboration with colleagues in other disciplines such as radiology and laboratory medicine.

- **Monday AM:** Ward round of inpatients and meet with the nurses, physiotherapists, occupational therapists and social services to discuss the further management of inpatients. Then meet with each patient on the ward round and explain to each patient their diagnosis and plans for future treatment.

  Monday lunchtime: I teach the foundation year 2 (F2) doctors on medical cases that they have seen or are looking after on the wards. Over a period of 6 months, we aim to cover most of the likely clinical presentations that a doctor is likely to see on the wards.

  Monday PM: Dictate letters to general practitioners about patients who have been discharged and review any laboratory reports on patients who have been seen in clinics.

- **Tuesday AM:** Medical outpatient clinic – three new patients who have been referred by their general practitioners with a variety of non-specific complaints for diagnosis and management. Depending on the complexity, it may take up to an hour to see, examine and plan future investigation and management. At the same time, trainee doctors are seeing other patients in the clinic and seek my advice on aspects of medical management.

  Tuesday lunchtime: Meet with junior doctors in the Medical Postgraduate Centre to discuss training issues and supervise organized teaching for the foundation programme doctors.

Tuesday PM: Medical ward round of medical inpatients (25–30 patients to be seen). Most of these patients will have been admitted as medical emergencies within the last week. There are a variety of clinical issues to be dealt with, including refining diagnoses, optimizing current treatments and planning patient discharge from hospital. At the end of the ward round, we go to see patients in other departments who have been referred for specific medical opinions.

Wednesday AM: Rehabilitation ward round. I am seeing patients who are recovering from strokes, falls and pneumonias. My team are on acute medical take, and are therefore seeing patients as they present to the medical admissions unit of the hospital.

Wednesday PM: Our take finishes at 4 PM, after which I do my post-take ward round, reviewing all the patients who have been seen by the team, while also providing teaching on each case to the junior members and medical students of the team. I return home at 8:30 PM.

Thursday AM: At 9 AM, meet with my team to discuss any new developments on patients since our medical take yesterday. At 9:30 AM, I am doing another outpatient clinic, more follow-ups of patients referred by their general practitioners and patients recently discharged from the medical wards. Luckily, most of the ward patients are making a good recovery, and so my job is made a little easier!

Thursday PM: Medical grand rounds. This is an opportunity to hear about interesting medical cases that have been seen by my colleagues in their clinical practice. The cases are discussed in the light of the latest medical evidence on the case. There is a lively debate among my colleagues as to the diagnoses and management of the case. I am always interested in the outcome, and consider how to apply this new-found knowledge to my future clinical practice.

We have our team X-ray meeting, where we discuss the X-rays or scans of each patient in consultation with a senior radiologist. Some diagnoses are changed and in some cases new tests are ordered. At 3 PM, I teach the medical students at the lecture theatre. The students present the cases they have seen themselves to me, and I provide feedback. I attend an administrative meeting at 4 PM to discuss management issues around how best to continue to provide the high standard of clinical care our patients have come to expect in an ever-changing NHS. At the end of the meeting, I return to the wards to review those patients who remain unwell following the acute admission yesterday.

Friday AM: Medical ward round with the final-year medical students and junior doctors. Most of the patients are getting better and some are able to go home, and plans on the patients' care are put in place for the coming weekend. At the end of the ward round, I teach some of the students clinical examination skills at the bedside. We contact the doctors who are going to look after the patients over the weekend and ensure that they are fully aware of the team's care plan for these patients should they deteriorate over the weekend.

Friday PM: I do another rehabilitation ward round and reassess patients who have become unwell during the week. I retire to my office for some routine administrative duties, particularly related to the on-call rota, junior doctors' leave and the teaching programme for the foundation programme doctor. I leave the hospital for home for a well-earned break for the weekend. Then back to work on Monday for another interesting and varied week in clinical medicine.

Ethical issues in modern medical practice

13

Professor Raanan Gillon, Emeritus Professor of Medical Ethics, Imperial College, London

This chapter will give an insight into ethical issues in modern medical practice, and will focus on how these issues can be approached.

Medical ethics

One of the skills you will need these days if you become a doctor is some knowledge of medical ethics and medical law, and an ability to think reasonably and critically about medical ethics issues in general. The GMC, which controls medical education and medical standards in the UK, has specified that medical ethics and law should be part of the core curriculum for medical students.[1] Some years ago, most medical school teachers of these subjects drew up a core curriculum outlining subjects that students should study during medical school.[2] So, as a medical student, you will have to come to know the main professional and legal obligations of doctors in the UK and to get to grips with the following ethically and legally important subjects:

- Informed consent and refusal of treatment.
- Truthfulness, trust and good communications in the doctor–patient relationship.
- Confidentiality and privacy.
- Medical research, its connections with ordinary therapeutic medical practice, and the special ethical and legal concerns relevant to it.
- A variety of ethical and legal aspects of human reproduction; for example, those associated with embryo research, in vitro fertilization and abortion.
- The 'new genetics'; for example, gene therapy, genetic testing and different forms of cloning.
- Treatment of children and issues such as children's rights, the relationship between age and competence to accept or refuse treatment, child abuse, and questions about decision-making on behalf of children.

- Mental illness and disorder and its associated ethical and legal problems; for example, compulsory treatment of some severely mentally disordered patients.

- Life-and-death issues, including debates about differences between allowing patients to die and killing them, euthanasia and physician-assisted suicide, what is meant by 'death' and 'brain death', and doctors' legal obligations in relation to death (a relatively mundane but in practice very important example is their legal duty to certify deaths).

- Resource allocation issues and questions of distributive justice: How might we fairly distribute scarce healthcare resources? How might we fairly 'ration' such resources? What are the pros and cons of different approaches, including those of different healthcare systems, to these questions?

- Rights, including human rights: What are they and what is their role in medical ethics and law?

- The vulnerabilities that the duties of doctors and medical students, and public expectations of them, create. Various issues that can have adverse effects on doctors and medical students also need ethical and legal exploration; for example, the need to be able to deal with uncertainty, various legal and professional regulations that apply to doctors, public expectations and concerns, ill health afflicting doctors and medical students themselves, and 'whistle-blowing' when a medical student or doctor believes something unethical and/or illegal is going on around him or her.

This is quite an extensive list of ethical and legal issues to think about over the few years of medical studies, not to mention over the course of your professional life if you become a doctor. For my own part as a doctor who studied philosophy in order to try and think more clearly about my ethical obligations, I have found the 'four principles plus scope' approach very helpful for ordering my thoughts and summarizing my medical ethical obligations.

'Four principles plus scope' approach

The four principles are:

1. Respect for autonomy
2. Beneficence
3. Non-maleficence
4. Justice.

The scope of applying such principles is also an important issue: To whom or to what do we owe these obligations? These principles do not provide a method of choosing the correct one when they conflict – they are prima facie and do not provide a set of ordered rules or an algorithm for moral judgements. That is where the elusive quality of good *judgement* comes in. However, the principles do provide a common set of moral commitments, a common moral language, and a common set of moral issues that can be used to help us reflect about the many ethical problems posed by medical practice and inform the necessary judgements.

Respect for autonomy

Autonomy can be thought of as 'deliberated self-rule'. Respect for autonomy is the moral obligation to respect the autonomy of a person insofar as such respect is compatible with equal respect for the autonomy of all potentially affected. In modern medical practice, this principle has many prima facie implications. It requires doctors to consult patients and give them adequate information and to obtain their consent before the patient can be helped and treated. It also requires doctors not to deceive patients – for example, not to deceive them about the diagnosis of their illness unless, of course, they do not wish to be told.

This principle even means that doctors, and other healthcare professionals, should be punctual for their appointments – an agreed appointment with a patient is a type of mutual promise, and arriving late or not keeping the appointment would be breaking the promise and, thus, not respecting the other person's autonomy.

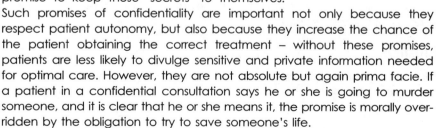

Medical confidentiality is another example of respecting the patient's autonomy. Patients tell doctors their symptoms, worries and other personal information in confidence, and doctors promise to keep these 'secrets' to themselves.

Such promises of confidentiality are important not only because they respect patient autonomy, but also because they increase the chance of the patient obtaining the correct treatment – without these promises, patients are less likely to divulge sensitive and private information needed for optimal care. However, they are not absolute but again prima facie. If a patient in a confidential consultation says he or she is going to murder someone, and it is clear that he or she means it, the promise is morally overridden by the obligation to try to save someone's life.

These are only a few examples of the prima facie obligations stemming from respect for the patient's autonomy in medical practice. For these to be carried out, doctors need to have good interpersonal skills and be good communicators. They should be good listeners and should be able to give the patient relevant information when they think appropriate (e.g. a run-through of treatment strategies currently available for their specific illness, suggesting the best, most suitable treatment option, and determining whether or not the patient would be interested in that particular option), as many patients choose to be involved in 'having a say' in and deciding their medical care. Others, however, do not want much information and prefer to leave the decision on their treatment to the doctor. Thus, doctors should try to ascertain the patient's needs and preferences for meeting them so that they can respect their autonomy.

Beneficence and non-maleficence

Beneficence means the act of doing good, and maleficence means doing harm. The traditional moral obligation in medicine, from Hippocratic times, is to provide optimal medical benefit to the patient with the least amount of harm, i.e. beneficence with non-maleficence. For this to be achieved, doctors should make sure that they can actually provide the benefits that they profess they can provide. They need to ensure that they have an effective education and training not only before they qualify but throughout their medical careers.

In order to offer every patient net benefit with minimal harm, the patient's own views should, where possible, be ascertained, as what may be a benefit to one patient may be harmful to another. Medical professionals should also be aware of any risks related to proposed healthcare interventions, and should really define at the outset who is likely to benefit from such interventions. This is particularly important in medical research, so as to avoid imposing risks greater than minimal on research subjects unless such risks are in the patient's own interests.

One moral concept that has become increasingly popular over recent years is helping patients to be more in control of and take an interest in their own health. This concept is known as 'empowerment'. It is a mixture of respecting patients' autonomy and beneficence, in the sense of helping them to understand how they can to some extent control and improve their own health.

Justice

Justice can briefly be defined as the moral obligation to act on the basis of fair adjudication between competing claims. When considering justice in medicine, there are three aspects of particular importance:

- distributive justice – fair distribution of scarce resources
- rights-based justice – respect for people's rights (including their human rights)
- legal justice – respect for morally acceptable laws.

Justice is not only about treating people equally. As Aristotle pointed out more than 2000 years ago, it is about treating equally those who ought to be treated equally and treating unequally those who ought to be treated unequally, and doing so in proportion to the morally relevant inequalities. For example, we should all be treated equally under the law; however, the law should treat us unequally (differently) if we deserve to be treated unequally. For instance, those guilty of an offence should be treated differently from those who have not committed an offence – that is part of legal justice.

In distributing scarce healthcare resources, we should treat people unequally in relation to morally relevant inequalities. For an obvious example, people with unequal healthcare needs should be treated unequally, with more resources going to those with greater needs. There are other potentially relevant criteria as well as need, such as the amount of benefit a unit of resource will provide both for an individual patient and for a population as a whole, the views of the persons in need (they may reject what they need), and the views of the people who provide the resources (e.g. taxpayers and their parliamentary representatives). We simply have not agreed on how to balance these conflicting moral values in a substantive theory of distributive justice (and we probably never will!). What we can, and, I believe, we should, do is avoid obviously unjust ways of distributing scarce resources (e.g. mere personal preference such as 'I like x better than y or racial, social or gender prejudice), and work within democratically established procedures for balancing or 'harmonizing' conflicting moral values. We should also be open about what those procedures are, and accept that it is inevitable that there will never be enough resources to enable all the moral values to be honoured all the time, or even to enable all needs to be met. So, even if allocation is entirely fair or just, it will inevitably be resented for not meeting all needs, and not honouring all conflicting moral concerns and claims at once.

Scope of applying the principles

Many important questions arise when the scope of applying the four principles is considered. For example, to whom do healthcare professionals have a duty of beneficence? To what extent should they be helped? Who or what falls into the scope of distributing resources fairly according to the principle of justice – only the people in a particular country or internationally?

As far as beneficence is concerned, doctors clearly owe this to all their patients. But what about people who are not patients yet are ill?

Who is to be included within the scope of the principle of respect of autonomy? Some patients are clearly not included within the scope of this principle because they are not autonomous at all. For example, newborn babies are not autonomous, as they are not able to deliberate. What about infants and young children, severely mentally ill people or the elderly with severe dementia? Will they be autonomous enough to make certain decisions, such as to have or refuse an operation? They may not be – but yet they may be able to decide what clothes to wear, which television programme they want to watch and which foods they want to eat. If such inadequately autonomous patients make decisions that seem, according to the doctor, to be against their interests, then issues such as who should make decisions on their behalf arise.

Another important scope issue is who and what has the 'right to life'? This issue remains highly controversial among healthcare professionals and in society generally. What is the right of life – the right to be kept alive or not to be unfairly killed? Who exactly has the right to life? Do non-humans (e.g. animals and plants) have this right? What about human embryos, fetuses and brain-dead patients – are they 'people' and do they have the right to life? People often think that disagreement about such issues demonstrates radical disagreement about moral values; however, it seems to me that the disagreement is instead metaphysical (concerning the nature of reality) and/or theological, although of course it has major moral consequences. Thus, we all agree that we should not murder each other. However, we may disagree profoundly about what we mean by 'each other' and, in particular, about whether or not an embryo or a fetus (or a brain-dead human being) falls within the scope of this obligation not to murder each other.

Summary

■ The 'four principles plus scope approach' provides a simple and accessible method for thinking about ethical issues in healthcare.

■ It allows doctors from completely different moral cultures to share a common moral commitment, a common moral language and a common analytical framework for reflecting on issues that arise at work.

■ This approach can be shared by everyone, regardless of their background, as it is culturally, philosophically and politically neutral.

References and further reading

1. General Medical Council. *Tomorrow's Doctors*. London: GMC, 1993: **14**, 26.

2. Teachers of medical ethics and law in UK medical schools. Teaching medical ethics and law within medical education: a model for the UK core curriculum. *J Med Ethics* 1998; **24**: 188–92.

Doyal L, Gillon R. Medical ethics and law as a core subject in medical education. A core curriculum offers flexibility in how it is taught – but not that it is taught. *BMJ* 1998; **316**: 1623–4.

Gillon R. *Philosophical Medical Ethics*. Chichester: Wiley, 1986.

Gillon R. Medical ethics: four principles plus attention to scope. *BMJ* 1994; **309**: 184–8.

An alternative career in medicine: Medical journalism

14

Dr Kamran Abbasi, *Editor*, Journal of the Royal Society of Medicine, *London*

This chapter discusses one of the more popular alternative or adjunct careers for medics, that of medical journalism. The author, who has been an acting editor of the *British Medical Journal (BMJ)* and is currently editor of the *Journal of the Royal Society of Medicine (JRSM)*, describes his own experiences and provides advice for those considering a career in medical journalism.

Among the tens of thousands of medical journals, only four are major weekly publications:

- *BMJ*
- *Lancet*
- *Journal of the American Medical Association (JAMA)*
- *New England Journal of Medicine.*

Working on these is as close as you can get (within the world of medical journals) to a newspaper, although medical journals are far more scholarly, polite and conservative publications.

What skills do I need?

The skills required to work on these journals are several. The most important of these is a sound judgement of what readers might or should be interested in reading. In addition, an ability to understand the clinical relevance of research and an appreciation and tolerance of differing perspectives are also vital.

One of the most valuable lessons I was ever taught was that journals are about debate and not about truth. Only rarely are opinions, even evidence-informed ones, absolute. There is likely to be a different interpretation and every chance that a future study will make the current dogma obsolete.

Sound critical appraisal and journalistic skills are also crucial, although do not worry if you are stronger in one area than the other. The large weekly journals not only commission, edit and write articles, but also offer opportunities to people who love reading and evaluating research papers.

Editors who are lucky enough to possess both of these attributes are likely to be particularly successful, as the best medical journals are now a mix of journalism and research.

To become the editor or deputy editor of one of the big UK journals, you will require all these skills plus the ability to manage people and preferably some business skills. Only a handful of people ever acquire the skills, opportunity or good fortune to become the editor of a major weekly medical journal, although the routes to the top differ between journals.

How do I start?

The *BMJ*, for example, offers an entry-level position, known as editorial registrar, which is a one-year training post for people with several years' experience of clinical medicine. The successful applicant usually displays some evidence of an interest in journalism and an aptitude for the intellectual challenges that an editorial position poses. A successful year as an editorial registrar is a gateway to a career in medical journalism, either at the *BMJ* or elsewhere. Another route into the *BMJ* is for medical students to apply for the post of editor of the *studentBMJ*, which is also essentially a training post in medical journalism, with the emphasis being more on journalism than science.

Occasionally, other editorial posts are advertised at the *BMJ* or the *Lancet* for people with a healthcare qualification, some clinical experience and a demonstrable interest in journalism. These are usually at the assistant editor level and may involve editing a section of the journal, peer review or a combination of the two. The *BMJ*, being clinically focused, tends to employ doctors as editors, apart from the few journalists who edit the purely journalistic news and reviews sections. The *Lancet*, in contrast, employs science graduates as well as medical graduates, reflecting its greater attention to basic science.

Another important difference between the *BMJ* and the *Lancet* is that at the *Lancet*, editors tend to take responsibility for research articles on specific topic areas, while *BMJ* editors do not usually have a particular area of specialist expertise. The *Lancet* does not have an equivalent training scheme to the *BMJ*'s editorial registrar post or student journal, but, like the *BMJ*, it is willing to consider applications from people who want to gain work experience on a weekly medical publication. You must be prepared for disappointment if you apply for any of these positions, because usually there are many applicants and there are only a few positions.

What is the training like?

The British model of weekly medical journals is based on a senior editor. He or she will have been trained for many years on the journal, and will no longer see themselves as a practising clinician or researcher but rather as a journalist first and a doctor second. Since editors tend to stay in post for many years, it can become quite a challenge to find development opportunities for doctors who are assistant editors on these journals and want to further their careers. Another thought to consider is that editors of junior or middling seniority are unlikely to match the pay of their colleagues working in hospital or general practice. However, for people who make their career on these journals, these concerns are outweighed by job security, a broader view of the world of medicine, and the thrill of being at the heart of developments in UK and international healthcare.

Although the *BMJ* and the *Lancet* may be the highest-profile medical journals in the UK, there are hundreds, possibly thousands, of so-called specialist journals. These offer an alternative route into the world of medical journalism. Usually, they are monthly publications, like *Gut*, *Thorax* and the *British Journal of General Practice*. Some are quarterly, and a few even less frequent. Another model is for online journals to offer publication of articles when they are ready and not really have a regular rhythm or specific issues.

The editors of these publications tend to be highly regarded clinicians in their specialties who have a passion for editing, but not necessarily any knowledge or experience. Some of these journals also employ associate editors who will look after a percentage of the research articles that have been submitted. The more progressive of these specialist journals are recognizing a move away from publishing only research articles and into publishing value-added material such as editorials, reviews and other educational content. Again, associate editors may be appointed to look after these specific sections.

Editors on these journals may have no experience in medical journalism but, being bright fellows, they quickly acquire the skills for their new role. Some, of course, find their whole tenure – which usually is a fixed term from 3 to 5 years – a struggle.

Being an editor

One attractive feature of an editorial post on a specialist journal is that you can continue with your full-time clinical commitment and also receive a salary for editing the journal. Apart from the financial benefit, the bigger gain is that your profile in your specialty will receive an immediate boost. The route to an editorial post on a specialist journal is usually to develop an impressive reputation in your specialty and your specialist society as a clinician and a researcher. In addition, it will help if you can demonstrate experience of peer review and writing for journals.

In comparison, the *JRSM* has become an unusual hybrid, being a monthly multispecialty journal. While editors previously were clinicians first and foremost, my predecessor Robin Fox, formerly editor of the *Lancet*, and I have both held senior posts on the *Lancet* and the *BMJ* respectively. The thinking is that even monthly journals will have to do more than just publish research to flourish in the age of the internet, and an experienced medical journalist and editor is more likely to develop a journal in a competitive market.

Non-medical journals

Medical journals are not the only opportunity for a career in medical journalism. Newspapers and magazines increasingly cover health issues, so there is scope for both doctors who want to abandon medicine and become health journalists and clinicians who want to be known as 'medical experts' to the unsuspecting public. The first of these options requires you to probably abandon your full-time career as a doctor and enter the murky and unpredictable world of freelance journalism.

Those interested in becoming a 'medical expert' for a newspaper or magazine will either have to become a doctor of such importance that they cannot be ignored or have the good fortune to be given such a title. Either way in lies uncertainty and a great deal of risk for most medical graduates. To standardize the procedure somewhat, some universities are now offering degree courses in medical journalism – and that might be a good way to test your resolve.

Whichever of these avenues you pursue, medical journalism is great fun if you can acquire enough skill and good fortune to find your way in.

Summary

- Medical journalism will continue to expand and offer opportunities for doctors with editorial and journalistic skills.
- A sound judgement of what readers might or should be interested in reading is required to write well.
- An ability to understand the clinical relevance of research and an appreciation and tolerance of differing perspectives are also vital.
- A successful year as an editorial registrar is a gateway to a career in journal-based medical journalism.
- Medical journal editors tend to be highly regarded clinicians in their specialties who have a passion for editing.

Academic medicine

15

Professor Robin Williamson, *Professor of Surgery, Imperial College London, Consultant Surgeon, Hammersmith Hospital and Emeritus Dean, Royal Society of Medicine, London*

What is entailed?

Academic medicine is usually taken to mean those aspects of a doctor's work that are distinct from looking after patients – namely research and teaching. Yet in practice these activities are not really distinct. Clinical research, for example, as opposed to laboratory research, involves trying out new treatments on patients, sometimes as an adjunct to existing methods and sometimes as an alternative. Most clinical teaching takes place at the bedside, in the outpatient clinic or in the operating theatre, and is therefore a natural extension of patient care. Therefore, academic medicine is more an attitude of mind than a separate part of the job. Good research requires some originality of thought – the ability to take a fresh look at the diagnosis or treatment of disease – and the commitment to translate ideas into practice. Good teaching requires enthusiasm, effort and empathy. These qualities are equally valuable in clinical medicine.

Who is involved?

Academic doctors are no more a separate species than academic medicine is divorced from clinical practice. Some of the most important discoveries in medicine have come not from a university department but from an 'ordinary' district general hospital, where a doctor has had the courage and determination to challenge dogma and try something new. Most clinical teaching is actually carried out by NHS consultants and junior staff, although true academics play a major role in arranging the undergraduate curricula and organizing the exams. By 'true academics' is meant doctors who work in a university department, the head of which is usually a professor. Medical schools in Britain will often have more than one professor in the main disciplines such as medicine, surgery, pathology, paediatrics and so on. Some of these will occupy most of their time with research, but the majority play an active part in patient care within the university hospital.

Academic medicine has a parallel career structure to 'service' medicine in the NHS. Much of the day-to-day research is carried out by trainees, whether research fellows or lecturers, who are roughly equivalent to the present clinical grades of senior house officer and registrar. Once an academic doctor reaches consultant rank (i.e. is capable of independent clinical practice), he or she becomes a senior lecturer with the potential for promotion on the academic ladder to reader or full professor. Professors are relatively scarce in Britain in comparison with many other countries, in which senior lecturers are called assistant professors and readers are called associate professors. However, their ranks have been swelled over recent years by appointments to 'satellite' academic units in university hospitals remote from the main medical school. The system is flexible – and correctly so. Many young doctors have a spell in a university department, where they develop an interest in research, but revert to the NHS at a later stage in their career to pursue their primary aim of looking after patients. Teaching hospitals often have on their staff men and women who were appointed as senior lecturers but have moved across to the NHS after a period of some years when a suitable vacancy arose. It is sometimes easier to obtain one's first consultant appointment in a university department where senior colleagues are available to provide some clinical support.

Advantages of academic medicine

Perhaps the main attraction of an academic appointment is the excitement that comes from innovation. This does not mean that a life devoted to looking after patients in hospital or the community is dull; on the contrary, it offers a constant challenge. Many doctors find complete fulfilment in patient care, particularly when the system allows them to pass on their knowledge and craft to those they are training. Yet, despite the phenomenal pace of medical advance, we remain ignorant about the cause and treatment of many diseases, and some doctors will relish the thrill that comes from research. Academic doctors are part-time clinicians to a greater or lesser extent. They have an extra dimension to their working week, with 'protected' time in the laboratory or office for study, research, writing, and the preparation of scientific papers or teaching materials. The protection will be relative, however, unless your research appointment is fulltime; a clinical problem can sometimes take you away from the bench. In some medical specialties, rotas can allow clinical academics to work one week on the ward and one week in the laboratory, but in 'service' disciplines such as surgery or obstetrics and gynaecology, such complete separation is seldom possible.

Academic medicine is not only fun; it can be seriously good for your career. In many popular fields of medicine, potential candidates outnumber training posts. Imagine you had to select one person from a group of 30 applicants, all of whom had the basic clinical qualifications for the job in question. You might set a good deal of store by interviews, but it would not be practicable to see every candidate. To draw up a shortlist, you would find yourself looking through each CV to find extra achievements that would distinguish one applicant from another. Academic medicine provides access to many of these achievements in the form of presentations to medical societies and publications in peer-reviewed journals. This is why many doctors, especially those ambitious for a teaching hospital consultant post, will take the time and trouble to do some research, write papers and perhaps obtain a higher degree such as an MD or PhD. The exercise itself can be surprisingly addictive. Many of those who submit to the rigours of research with the prime objective of advancing their career find themselves drawn into the thrill of the chase. After a year or two of research, you have probably become a world expert in a small field of medicine. Some find this experience so satisfying that they devote the rest of their lives to research. Others go back to clinical medicine, but retain the capacity for independent thinking and critical assessment of other people's work. Almost all benefit from the experience, both intellectually and practically.

There are other tangible rewards for the hours spent on the laboratory bench doing an experiment or on laptop composition. Academic activities add variety to a working life. If the clinical going is tough, you can beaver away at the bench. If the experiment fails, you can concentrate for a while on looking after real people on the ward. Medical conferences become a feature of your life, and they are frequently held in interesting places. You meet research workers and fellow enthusiasts from other cities and countries who become firm friends after repeated encounters. Anyone with a bent for travel will enjoy the international conference scene, and it actually counts as work! Academic doctors are often invited to act as visiting lecturers and examiners in Britain and abroad, and this provides another chance to brush up on your geography as well as your diplomacy and presentational skills.

It is only as I approach retirement that I have come to appreciate how many different openings medicine can offer throughout a working life. In this respect, experience of academic medicine is a useful attribute (though by no means essential). You could gravitate towards a career in either university or NHS administration, ending as a vice-chancellor or a member of a Trust board, or become an officer of a Royal College, or remain a practising clinician or scientist with an international reputation. In the game of life, academic medicine provides an additional qualification.

Disadvantages of academic medicine

You may have set off to become a practising doctor only to be derailed by the fascination of research and spend the rest of your life at the bench. Is this a disadvantage though? Probably not: it is more likely that you have stumbled across the best outlet for your talents. Of course, not all research goes swimmingly. Three-quarters of the way through my year in a laboratory in Boston, I found that someone had just published the very experiment that I was performing. After my heart had sunk to the bottom, I reread the paper and found that I had not really been scooped; there were so many flaws in design and interpretation that it strengthened my own chance to contribute to the field. If a medical experiment addresses an important question in an appropriate manner, the result will be of value, even if negative.

There may be some financial sacrifices to be made in an academic life. Doctors working in certain branches of medicine, orthopaedic surgery, for example, may be able to double their salary or more from private practice, and this opportunity is denied (or at least restricted) for academics. Incidentally, it is sometimes forgotten that private practice is very hard work, coming on top of NHS responsibilities and undertaken in the evenings and at weekends. Those who rise to the top of the academic tree may receive some financial compensation from the clinical excellence awards that are available for doctors who make additional contributions to the health service, but that requires a major involvement in clinical work.

Academic doctors can find it difficult to serve two masters: the university, which is generally the employer, and the NHS, which provides the clinical facilities. Each expects a pretty full commitment, and each will have its own appraisal process. Academics tend to be judged on their ability to obtain research grant funding as well as their productivity in terms of scientific papers; excellence in teaching does not always attract the credit it deserves. The hospital authorities naturally expect those with an honorary contract to honour their clinical responsibilities (including on-call duties), and these need to be balanced against the demands of academic life.

Getting started

It is never too early to become involved in academic medicine. Most undergraduate courses include the opportunity to undertake a period of research, either as an intercalated year towards a BSc, BMedSci degree or sometimes in a modular course interspersed with clinical attachments. In this way, some students will have a publication to their name even before they qualify as a doctor. Postgraduate medical training is changing fast with the government's directive on Modernising Medical Careers, but it seems likely that the second foundation year (starting one year after graduation) will include the possibility of an academic attachment. Do not despair if this opportunity does not occur: there are plenty of chances to get into academic medicine at a later stage of training. Professors in every medical discipline are always on the lookout for those with an aptitude and enthusiasm for research, and will welcome enquiries from doctors with a potential interest. It may be best to delay starting a formal research project until you have determined your major career pathway, but it is not essential; many laboratory techniques are applicable to a wide range of medical specialties.

Why not give academic medicine a try? It could revolutionize your career, as it did mine. If it does not, you have lost very little. A spell in an academic department will sharpen up your critical faculties and give you a respect for innovation and communication that can hardly fail to make you a better doctor.

Some popular misconceptions

- *'Those who can, do; those who cannot, teach.'* This tired old cliché certainly does not apply to clinical medicine. The best teachers are those who are actively practising their subject, whether patient care or laboratory research.

- *'Academics inhabit an ivory tower remote from the cut-and-thrust of everyday patients.'* I have tried to show that academic doctors do most of what other NHS doctors do, but, in addition, spend part of their week engaged in teaching and research. They are certainly not missing out on the demands or the satisfaction of looking after sick people. Instead, they have an extra avenue for potential fulfilment.

- *'Research is glamorous.'* Occasionally it is, but eureka moments are scarce. Much research is a hard slog, and success cannot often be measured in the short term. Sometimes your published finding lies dormant until you or someone else makes a new discovery that demonstrates the importance of the original work.

- *'I might embark on an academic career and then run out of ideas for anything new.'* Perhaps – but this is seldom the case. A well-conducted experiment tends to throw up half a dozen new avenues for fruitful exploration. As academic doctors become more senior, however, their contribution widens to providing facilities for research and supervising others rather than just carrying out 'hands-on' experiments. With reasonable luck, your first experience of research will be gained with the help of someone who can give you the necessary help to get under way.

■ *'I might get trapped at a laboratory bench and miss out on the chance of becoming a "proper" doctor.'* This is untrue: no one need feel trapped. There is a free, two-way flow between academic medicine and service medicine, with the ability to switch horses at almost any stage. Most people find a period of academic activity rewarding both intellectually and practically in terms of career development.

■ *'Publish or die.'* It is true that those engaged in research need to publish their findings, but quality is more important than quantity. Since all research costs money, it is important to show that the time and effort have been well spent. Fortunately, there is a huge array of medical journals with editors eager to publish work that has been sensibly conducted and clearly explained. The conduct and writing up of an experiment are skills that can readily be learned.

Index